Fast Migraine Headache Relief With EFT Tapping

Relief is a close as your fingertips!

Brad Reed

www.WithEFTtapping.com

Copyright Notice

Copyright © 2013 Brad Reed and Transformation Bay, LLC. All rights reserved.

Reproduction or translation of any part of this work beyond that permitted by section 107 or 108 of the 1976 United State Copyright Act without permission of the copyright owner is unlawful. Request for permission or further information should be addressed to the author.

Brad Reed, Transformation Bay LLC.

www.WithEFTtapping.com

This publication is designed to provide accurate and authoritative information in regard to the subject matter covered. It is sold with the understanding that the author and publisher are not engaged in rendering medical, legal, accounting, or other professional services. If medical, legal or other advice or expert assistance is required, the services of a competent professional person should be sought.

All photos are Copyright © 2013 Brad Reed

Cover design Copyright © 2013 Brad Reed

Part of the cover design is presented as a derivative work based on licensed material which is © iStockphoto.com/fredgoldstein

First printing, 2013.

ISBN-13: 978-1494289874
ISBN-10: 1494289873

Printed in the United States Of America.

Disclaimers

The information, instructions, and advice contained in this publication are for educational purposes only. Brad Reed, and Transformation Bay LLC, and the content of this publication cannot be relied upon as treatment, cure, or for prevention of any medical condition, disease, or life situation. It is recommended that you consult with a qualified medical practitioner before acting on or implementing any of the information or recommendations made in this publication. Any use of the information contained in this publication is at your own risk. Because there is always some risk associated with and involved in making life and health changes, Brad Reed, and Transformation Bay LLC are not responsible for any consequences or adverse effects of any kind resulting from the use or misuse of any information, instructions, suggestions, or advice described in this publication. The information is provided "as is" without any representations or warranties, expressed or implied. The reader and/or possessor of these materials assume all risk from non-use, misuse, or use of this information.

The information presented in this publication represents the views of the author at the time of publication. Because conditions change and new information is published or revealed frequently, the author reserves the right to update or alter his opinion based on the new information and conditions. While best efforts have been used in preparing the information in this publication, the author assumes no responsibility for errors, inaccuracies, or omissions. Any slights of people or organizations are unintentional.

Affiliate Link Disclaimer

Please assume that any links in this document are affiliate links. If you were to purchase through one of these links I may receive some compensation for that purchase.

Some of the links in this document may go directly to the products and/or services that I offer, or that are offered as part of my business under Transformation Bay LLC or other businesses with which I have association.

The included affiliate links are for products and services that I have used, or come recommended by sources I personally trust. While I cannot vouch for any product or service that I have not personally created or deliver, there are many excellent products and services of which I am aware and have confidence in and thus feel comfortable recommending.

In the event that you do not wish to purchase through these affiliate links, you may use other means to locate these products or services through your favorite search engine on the web. I appreciate your support through the use of these affiliate links, but it is not required.

Table of Contents

Disclaimers v

Affiliate Link Disclaimer...vi

Introduction 1

    Why this matters.. 2

    What you'll learn... 3

    Why listen to me? 4

    Online Resources 5

How To Use This Book.. 7

Section 1: EFT Tapping.. 9

    Disclaimer 10

    Origins of EFT 11

    How does EFT work? 13

Overview of the EFT process 13

Choosing an issue to work on..13

Choosing a "summary description or label" for it 14

SUDS...16

Forming The Setup Phrase 16

The Setup 17

Tapping Process 19

Tapping Locations 20

EFT Protocol 22

Summary of basic steps for EFT Tapping 24

EFT Tapping Examples 25

Craving Demo... 26

Breathing Demo 31

Online video example.. 36

Troubleshooting Tips For Common Difficulties In Applying EFT Tapping 37

    Being too general 37

    Losing track of the issue.. 38

    Say it like it is so you can address the actual issue...................... 38

    Skipping steps.. 38

    Addressing an undefined or poorly specified issue...................... 39

    EFT Tapping on a Page 40

Section 2: Applying EFT Tapping For Fast Migraine Headache Relief 41

    How to use this section... 41

    If a Migraine Headache is starting now....................................... 42

    If you don't have Migraine symptoms right now.......................... 42

Getting Started With Migraine Headache EFT Tapping..................... 43

    Using SUDS, Character, and Location to guide your tapping process 43

Example Tapping Script Walk-Through 44

SUDS, Character, & Location – Initial Assessment 45

Setup Phrase and KC tapping 45

Tapping through the points 46

SUDS, Character, & Location reassessment 47

It shifted 47

Tapping through the points – Round 2 48

SUDS, Character, & Location reassessment after round 2 48

It didn't change - so what happened? 49

Tapping through the points – Round 3 49

SUDS, Character, & Location reassessment after round 3 50

Important things to watch for... 51

Focus on the feeling 51

Add Setup Phrase 51

EFT On A Page Cheat Sheet Migraine Edition 52

Migraine Tapping Fast Start 53

Using EFT Tapping To Address Migraine Triggers 59

Recognizing triggers 59

Physical Triggers 60

Emotional triggers 61

Stress 61

Anticipation induced stress 63

People, Anger, Power & Control 64

Tapping for triggers 65

The power of persistence 66

Tapping Frequently Asked Questions 67

Do I need to check with my Doctor before I start using EFT Tapping? 67

Who can use EFT Tapping? 68

Is it safe for kids to use EFT Tapping? 68

Is it safe to use EFT Tapping for other things? 68

Which side do I tap on – Right or Left? 69

How hard do I tap? 69

When should I start tapping? 69

How long should I tap? 70

How often should I tap? 70

How do I know that it's working? 71

What should I do when I notice a shift? 71

I noticed an initial shift, but now I'm stuck 72

What should I do if I don't notice a shift? 74

How do I know when I'm "done" tapping? 77

How can I be even more effective with EFT Tapping? 78

21-Ways To Get Even Better Results… 79

Frequently Asked Questions For Migraine Headaches 81

It hurts so bad that I don't want to physically tap, is there another way? 81

My child's pain is so intense that they won't let me help by tapping on them. Is there another way to help them with EFT? 82

Other Headache Tips And Tricks… 85

Base of the skull tapping 85

"Headache Point" on the hand 86

Section 3: Tips, Tricks, And Secrets For Using EFT Tapping 89

Floor-To-Ceiling Eye Roll Shortcut 89

Finger Tapping Points 91

Mental Tapping 92

Public tapping without embarrassment 93

Free Online Resources 93

Tapping Journal 94

Saying it like it is: Be politically INcorrect with your phrasing 95

Tap-And-Bitch 97

Borrowing Benefits 99

Conclusion 101

Resources 103

Videos 103

Downloadable EFT Tapping Cheat Sheets 104

Scholarly Research	104
From the Author, Brad Reed	104
Other Resources	105

Please leave a review of this book on Amazon.com 105

About the Author 107

Introduction

The world has Kristen Eckstein to thank for this book. If it were not for the fact that she was getting a Migraine Headache that September day in Baltimore back in 2010, I would have never had the opportunity to help her relieve those symptoms with EFT Tapping! Kristen was the very first person I helped to get fast relief from her Migraine Headache symptoms. While I didn't actually time how long it took, it certainly felt like it was only about four or five minutes before the symptoms were pretty much gone in her estimation. While I can't guarantee or even suggest that you will be able to achieve those kinds of results, I can tell you that I've done my best to include in this book all the information you need to learn how to apply EFT Tapping to Migraine Headache symptoms.

EFT Tapping is used throughout the world on a daily basis by tens of thousands of individuals to create a better life for themselves. Whether they are focused on using EFT Tapping to eliminate the pain of a Migraine Headache, eliminate their fear of heights, or helping a child get over their pain and sadness about being bullied at school, the results that are commonly delivered by this powerful tool are often nothing short of amazing. It doesn't matter if you are well versed in using EFT tapping and are looking for a new approach to dealing with Migraine Headache symptoms, or are brand new to EFT Tapping and this is your first exposure to it, you are in the right place.

I give you my personal promise that I will do my very best to provide you with valuable information that you can apply immediately in your life, and especially to Migraine symptoms. I use Tapping nearly every day, and there are even some days where I apply it multiple times during the day. While we never really know what challenges or upsets we may face during the day, by knowing how to apply EFT Tapping to the things that do happen in our lives we can release the pain, upset, and personal blocks that hold us back from living our full potential. You should consider yourself one of the lucky few who have found this material, because I know that for me, life without EFT Tapping would be far more painful and difficult every day.

Why this matters...

We can't always control what happens to us during the day. We do our best to plan and create the life that we desire, but there are times where the old joke, "Want to make God laugh? Tell him your plans!" really seems to apply. No one ever plans to have a genuine, full-blown Migraine on Tuesday afternoon at 3PM, but sometimes it just shows up anyway. The best thing that we can do is to learn the tools and strategies that will help us to cope and thrive in life. EFT Tapping is the best tool that I've ever found for creating a shift in my situation, regardless of what the situation may be. It is also the best tool that I'm aware of for shifting Migraine Headache pain in many cases.

Introduction

You may have plans for a romantic weekend…or at least you did before the Migraine Headache symptoms started. By knowing and applying the information contained in this book, you will likely be able to create a much more pleasant experience the next time it happens because you will know how to use EFT Tapping to help eliminate the Migraine symptoms before they ruin the weekend.

One of the most powerful reasons this matters is because with EFT Tapping relief can be as close as your fingertips. This is especially compelling because you can start applying this drug-free technique at the very first signs or inkling of Migraine symptoms. You don't have to wait until the symptoms are intense enough to prod you into taking some medication or applying the other techniques you use to try to get some Migraine symptom relief. EFT Tapping for Migraine Headaches is often the most effective when applied at the first sign of symptoms. While no one can absolutely guarantee results with EFT Tapping, or any other modality for that matter, it is one of the fastest and easiest to start applying when symptoms do show up.

I encourage you to read through this book carefully and actively participate in the EFT Tapping exercises that are included. You don't have to wait until Migraine symptoms are present to practice applying the technique. Practicing EFT Tapping before symptoms occur will get you familiar with this simple process so you are more fully prepared to use it when the need arises.

What you'll learn…

The first thing you'll learn is that I'm not a doctor, so you need to consult with a qualified medical practitioner before applying anything that you read in this book. The content presented here is for informational purposes and is NOT medical advice of any kind. Please do not proceed any further until you have read and understand the Disclaimer section at the beginning of this book.

The first section of this book will teach you the basics of EFT Tapping and how to apply it with the intention to create a shift within you. That shift may be the reduction or elimination of the pain of a Migraine Headache or even of a physical injury. The shift could also be the reduction or elimination of a fear that affects your ability to live life fully – like the fear of heights, or fear of flying. It could also be an internal shift that is sometimes more challenging to quantify, as when your attitude or outlook shifts, for example when you release your emotional upset or sadness around an event in your personal history. I've personally used EFT Tapping to release the sadness around the passing of my pet cat that I was particularly close to and had been missing terribly for a long time.

The second section of this book will show you how to use EFT Tapping to address the focus topic of this book – relieving Migraine Headache symptoms quickly. In this case, not only will you find a tapping script that you can follow along with, but you will also find a number of suggestions on how to be even more effective in applying EFT Tapping toward Migraine Headache relief. This section also includes information on ways to apply EFT Tapping in your life to possibly help reduce the chances of having a Migraine Headache in the first place.

Why listen to me?

I decided to create this series of EFT Tapping books because I've personally seen too many people be negatively affected by the topics I cover. The amount of

Introduction

pain and suffering that I've seen in the world that could potentially be quickly and easily shifted with these techniques drives me to get these tools into the hands of as many people as I can.

For more than a decade, I've been teaching people how to use EFT Tapping to help them with physical symptoms like Migraines, eliminate self-sabotage, and clear away the roadblocks that are keeping them from success in many areas of their life.

I've been so successful with EFT that one of my case studies on fear of flying was even listed on the official EFT web site.

I'm so dedicated to thoroughly understanding EFT for myself, that not only have I studied the DVD training materials created by Gary Craig, the founder of EFT, and attended three of his live, in-person multi-day workshops, but I have invested the time, effort, and money to earn my EFTCert-1 through the only certification program recommended by Gary shortly before his retirement.

I'm not willing to settle for the uncertain quality and accuracy of "hand me down EFT" and you shouldn't be either. But if you are not able to learn directly from "the source" you should at least learn from someone who has!

Online Resources

Throughout this book are links to online resources. The links send you to a common landing page where the individual resources are available directly on that page, or as links to other pages. This way, as the content available on the internet changes and evolves, you will have access to the most up-to-date version. You will also have an opportunity there to sign up for access to updates, enhancements, and other bonus material.

How To Use This Book

If you are new to EFT Tapping then I would recommend that you read this book from cover to cover. It will give you a thorough understanding of the basics of EFT Tapping and how to apply it. In the future, when you need to do some more tapping, then you can simply refer to the summary information at the end of the chapters to refresh your memory, as well as revisit any specific steps or details that you want to clarify in your mind.

In addition, I would recommend looking at the resources section for other books in this series that are designed to address specific issues that you may also have need for as well. You may also find that there are topics covered that may not apply directly to you but may be helpful to a friend or loved one. Your personal recommendation can have a very powerful effect in helping them and on creating an even better life for themselves.

If you are familiar with EFT Tapping then I would recommend that you start by scanning through the first section of this book so that you are familiar with the specific vocabulary that I use and the way that I communicate the information.

Next, you can dig into the content dealing with Migraine Headaches in section 2. That is where the meat of this book will be for people already familiar with EFT Tapping.

If you have other EFT Tapping books in this series then you are certainly already familiar with EFT Tapping as I present it here. I would still recommend that you start by scanning through the first section of this book, because as I create additional members of this book series, I may add specific content for the topic as well as refine the way that I communicate the information.

Next, dig into section 2 where you will find the migraine-headache-specific content of this book. There you will find the information you are seeking on how to use EFT Tapping to address Migraine symptoms and create the relief you are after.

Section 1: EFT Tapping

What is EFT? EFT stands for Emotional Freedom Technique.

It can be likened to Emotional Acupuncture without needles. It has also been described as a form of acupressure, combined with mental focusing. It's really just a simple form of stress-reduction technique based upon the traditional Chinese energy meridian system - the same meridian system that's been used for the last 5000 years or so in acupuncture. The fact that they've been using it for SO long tells me that it must be effective or they would have abandoned it long ago.

EFT uses the same "energy meridian system" that is used in Acupuncture, but instead of using needles, you tap on specific energy meridian points on the body with your fingers. Whereas Acupuncture is often primarily focused on physical ailments, EFT is usually focused on the emotional side of things. But the cool part about EFT is that often times by "clearing" the "stuck energy" around the emotional side of things, the physical side will also improve dramatically. Many people use EFT to directly address physical issues by focusing on the thoughts, feelings, and emotions around the physical issue.

Disclaimer

Before we get started, I have to provide you with the following disclaimer (in addition to the one earlier in the book!):

- I'm not a doctor - I don't even play one on TV.
- The content presented here is for informational purposes only.
- The ideas, techniques, and suggestions presented here are not intended as a substitute for consulting with a professional health care provider.
- While many people have gotten great results using EFT, it's still considered an experimental modality.
- If you have any questions about whether or not to use EFT, please consult with your physician or licensed mental health practitioner.
- Do not discontinue any medication or treatment program without a doctor's supervision.
- You need to take responsibility for yourself - I can't take responsibility for, nor be held responsible for, you and your choices. Only you can do that.
- EFT is a registered trademark of its founder Gary Craig.
- Gary has retired and "Given EFT to the world" but he has no connection with, nor influence on, the content presented here.

- This is my version of EFT, which is based on all of the training I've had, from both Gary Craig and others.

Origins of EFT

Gary Craig, a Stanford University trained engineer, created EFT in about 1993 based on the principles he learned from Dr. Roger Callahan, a classically trained clinical psychologist. It was Dr. Callahan who made the original discoveries that laid the foundation upon which today's tapping modalities are built.

Dr. Callahan was working with a patient of his named Mary. She had an INTENSE water phobia since she was an infant. Water was so terrifying to her that she couldn't even take a bath in a tub full of water! She was even terrified each time it rained, and she had nightmares about "water getting her."

Dr. Callahan had been using conventional psychotherapy techniques with her for 18 months with virtually no progress. The best they had been able to achieve was to have Mary dangle her legs in the water on the edge of his swimming pool and not look at the water. At the end of each session she left with a terrible headache due to the stress.

Frustrated with their lack of progress, Dr. Callahan was looking outside of conventional means and had been studying the Acupuncture Energy Meridians. Mary had repeatedly mentioned that water gave her an awful feeling in the pit of her stomach. Dr. Callahan decided to try an experiment and asked Mary to tap on the end of the stomach meridian, which is directly under the eyes.

Much to his astonishment, Mary said, "It's gone! That horrible feeling I get in the pit of my stomach when I think about water is completely gone!" At first, he didn't believe her, but then she jumped up and ran toward the pool with no fear. Dr. Callahan was concerned because she couldn't swim, but Mary reassured him that even though the fear was gone, she knew she couldn't swim, it didn't make her stupid.

From there, Dr. Callahan went on to develop the technique further, and after a number of additional discoveries and tests with other patients, he developed Thought Field Therapy, or TFT. The method he created included some diagnostic steps and various tapping "recipes," that differed based on what the presenting problem was for that patient. He created a number of recipes that he used successfully with a variety of patients and conditions. He has successfully helped many people with other phobias, fears, and life-induced traumas as well.

Years Later, Gary Craig took some training from Dr. Callahan on the tapping method he had created. Through the eyes of a Stanford University trained engineer, Gary saw ways to simplify and generalize the TFT procedure, with its complex diagnostic steps and tapping "recipes", into a much simpler form of tapping that is now known as EFT, or Emotional Freedom Technique.

While there are many variations, and customizations that are cousins of EFT, they generally all fall under the generic term of Tapping Modalities. Whatever their variations may be, they all work with the same thing - the body's energy meridian system.

How does EFT work?

While there are a number of theories and explanations that have been put forth as to how EFT works, no one is really certain. Gary did come up with a workable explanation in The EFT Thesis statement, which is...

The cause of all negative emotion is a disruption in the body's energy system.

No one is really certain of how it works, but one thing is certain: tens of thousands of people use tapping every day and get great results!

Overview of the EFT process

The EFT process itself is made up of several simple steps:

- The first, you choose an incident, a feeling, a behavior, or a limitation to be addressed - You want to be very specific and focused on the feeling.
- Then you rate the intensity of the feeling, on a scale from 0-10, and note it for comparison later,
- Next you do the "Setup" and "Tap on it" using the EFT procedure,
- Then you rate the intensity again and decide if you need to repeat the tapping process in order to reduce the intensity even more.

Choosing an issue to work on

There are all kinds of things you could choose to address with EFT, even beyond Migraine Headache symptoms. (For the purpose of teaching EFT, I am using non-migraine examples in this section. Later in this book there is lots of information on how to apply EFT Tapping to Migraines.)

The key is to be specific about the details and feelings being addressed. You need to break down the issue into its component parts and address each one individually for maximum effectiveness.

For example, a "Fear of Flying" has many components or aspects - things like...

- Claustrophobia
- Fear of Heights
- Not Being in Control
- Leaving the Ground
- The feeling of turbulence
- Even the smells associated with aircraft and jet engine exhaust...

...may all contribute to the larger set of feelings given the label "Fear of Flying."

The idea is that after you break it down into its component parts, then you start by working on the individual component that has the highest level of intensity or discomfort.

Choosing a "summary description or label" for it

Some issues have long descriptions. It is valuable to figure out the long description so that you can "tune-in" to all the details of the exact issue. This would be an example of the "long description" of the issue.

"That time in the third grade when I was reading out loud in front of the class and I said the wrong word and I felt embarrassed because everyone laughed at me."

That would completely and accurately describe the issue you are focused on for tapping.

However, using the long description would be cumbersome during the tapping process. So we create a "summary description or label" to use as a shorthand way to represent the issue while we are tapping. The "shorthand" is used during the setup process to represent the entire issue for tapping. And it is also used during the tapping process to stay focused on the issue, as we defined it for this round of tapping. You can choose whatever "summary description or label" you want, but the point is to build one that represents the issue for YOU so you can stay focused on THAT issue.

For the previous example, there are several ways I could create a shorthand for it. I could say, "Reading out loud embarrassment" if that was the most important part for me. Or I could say, "Class laughed at me in the 3rd grade" if that was the key part. And notice I said "in the 3rd grade" because there may have been other times that the class laughed at me, but I want to focus on that particular incident in the 3rd grade. Another way would be "Wrong word, reading out loud" - it doesn't have to be grammatically correct or even complete.

Each of those phrases may actually represent a different aspect of the overall issue itself. Sometimes you may have to apply EFT to several aspects of an issue in order to get substantial emotional relief from the issue.

The idea of the "summary description or label" is to have something that represents the issue FOR YOU in order to stay focused on THAT issue and not accidentally switch to another issue without noticing it. The shorthand basically helps keep you focused on the item being addressed, rather than mentally jumping to similar items that may come to mind. And similar items OFTEN do come to mind in the middle of tapping. Simply make a mental note of them but finish the current round of tapping using the original focus for that round of tapping. The "new" items can be addressed with a separate round of tapping if needed.

SUDS

It is useful to measure the intensity of the item being addressed so that you can more easily notice the change resulting from the tapping process. In order to do that, we measure the intensity before tapping, and then again after tapping. We measure it by giving it a SUDS rating.

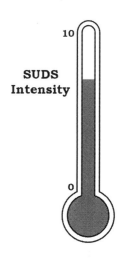

SUDS stand for Subjective Units of Distress Scale. It is an arbitrary 0 to 10 scale with 0 being no intensity and 10 being as intense as you can imagine it being

Forming The Setup Phrase

The first step to releasing an issue is to acknowledge it! While this may seem obvious, there is also a trick to it that many people don't realize.

You see, through no fault of your own, sometimes there is a degree of "Subconscious Self Sabotage" that is operating below the surface, unrecognized and unseen. That is because sometimes there is a subconscious part of you that is resistant to getting over an issue. That subconscious part may think it's not "safe" to get over the issue, because it sees that actually having the issue is protecting you in some way. And sometimes that subconscious part of you may think there is a secondary gain from actually having an issue.

For example, let's say you had a back injury and as a result you were getting disability payments. There could be a subconscious part of you that believes that if you were to get over your back injury, you would lose your disability payments. As a result, it doesn't feel it would be "safe" to get over the injury, so it is resistant to letting it go. And while it might be accurate that you could lose the disability payments, in fact that subconscious part would also be missing out on your conscious understanding of how much your life would improve by getting over the back injury, and getting your life back - even if you do have to go out and get a new job.

This scenario, and many more, fall under the heading of "Psychological Reversal." EFT has a specific way of addressing "Psychological Reversal," or PR, in order to improve the probability of success, and that is by doing the "setup process" before actually starting the tapping.

The Setup

The purpose of the Setup is to help get rid of any "psychological reversal" that may be associated with the issue. The Setup consists of tapping on the Karate Chop spot on the side of the hand, while saying a specific "Setup

Phrase."

The "Karate Chop" spot or KC is on the side of the hand between the base of the little finger and the wrist. It is where your hand would strike an object with a "Karate Chop." It doesn't matter which hand you tap on, but I always tap on it with the four fingers of the other hand.

The intention of the "Setup Phrase" is to let the subconscious know that "even though you have the problem or issue, you really are OK." And by letting the subconscious know that you're OK even though you have the problem, it is much more likely to "get out of the way" and allow the tapping to have its desired effect.

The format of the Setup Phrase is: "Even though {problem statement} I deeply and completely love and accept myself." In this case the {problem statement} can be a short description of the problem or I will often use the "summary description or label" we talked about earlier.

One of the key things to remember is to be as specific as possible in defining the issue that you're going to be addressing.

So to do the setup process you would tap on Karate Chop spot while saying the Setup Phrase out loud...

"Even though {problem statement} I deeply and completely love and accept myself."

Repeat Setup Phrase three times while tapping continuously on the Karate Chop Spot.

So if we were to be addressing the issue we discussed before, it could be done like this:

While tapping continuously on the Karate Chop spot, repeat out loud three times -

"Even though the class laughed at me in the 3rd grade, I deeply and completely love and accept myself."

"Even though the class laughed at me in the 3rd grade, I deeply and completely love and accept myself."

"Even though the class laughed at me in the 3rd grade, I deeply and completely love and accept myself."

You can say either, "I deeply and completely love and accept myself," or just, "I deeply and completely accept myself." Either one can be effective in letting the subconscious know that you're OK.

Sometimes people are REALLY resistant to saying, "I deeply and completely love and accept myself." What I recommend is to change it to, "I'm open to the possibility of deeply and completely loving and accepting myself...someday!" Usually people who run into that difficulty can be "open to the possibility...."

The other thing I recommend doing is to spend some time tapping on: "Even though I can't say that I deeply and completely love and accept myself, I deeply and completely love and accept myself anyway...or at least I'm open to that possibility someday!"

Tapping Process

The tapping is done on specific points on the body while saying the "Reminder Phrase" to keep you "tuned in" to the issue being addressed. The Reminder Phrase is the "summary description or label" that we talked about earlier. The points are bilateral, on both sides of the body, or on the center line of the body and correspond to specific acupuncture points. You can tap on either side of the body, or you can tap on both sides, which is what I usually do. I generally tap with two fingers at a time because it covers more area and I don't have to be as accurate on hitting THE spot. I generally tap about seven times on each spot or about as long as it takes to say the Reminder Phrase. The tapping pressure should be soft but firm - about as hard as you would press on a computer keyboard when typing.

Tapping Locations

There are nine specific spots that we are going to be tapping on as shown in the diagram below.

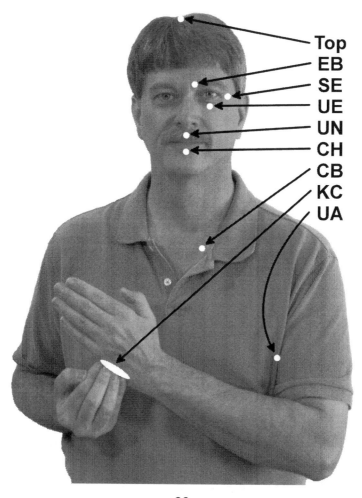

They are:

- The "Top" or Top of the Head.
- The "EB or Eyebrow at the end closest to the bridge of your nose.
- The "SE" or Side of the Eye - on the bony ridge beside the eye, NOT farther back on the softer temple area.
- The "UE" or Under the Eye spot on the bony ridge in line with the center of your eye.
- The UN or Under the Nose...is under the nose.
- The CH or "Chin Spot" is the next one. It is called the "Chin spot" but it is really under the lower lip.
- The CB or Collar bone is the next spot. You can find this by taking your finger and placing it on your "Adam's Apple" and then dropping down into the little U-shaped area at the base of your throat. Then move down and out about an inch and you should be on the collarbone next to where it meets the sternum or breastbone.
- The UA or Under Arm spot is on your side about 4 inches, or "a hand's width" below the arm pit.
- And we've already talked about the KC or "Karate Chop" spot which is on the side of the hand between base of little finger and wrist.

As an enhancement to this book, I created a video showing the tapping locations more clearly than can be done with words photos alone. You can see the EFT Tapping Locations video here:

http://tapping4.us/tappingspots

You can find a complete list of videos and other internet content in the Resources section.

Now that we know where we are going to be tapping, let's look at the actual EFT tapping protocol.

EFT Protocol

The first thing to do is to choose what issue to address, and give that issue an initial 0-10 SUDS rating.

Then begin by tapping on Karate Chop spot while saying the Setup Phrase out loud, three times.

"Even though {problem statement} I deeply & completely love & accept myself."

Next, tap through the sequence while saying the "Reminder Phrase" as you are tapping on each point. Tap on the Eyebrow, then Side of the Eye, Under the Eye, Under the Nose, Chin, Collar Bone, Under the Arm, and finally Top of the Head.

I recommend doing two or more rounds of tapping at a time

Once you've completed a couple of rounds of tapping, take a deep breath, and then give the issue a new SUDS rating.

Finally, compare the two SUDS ratings, which will determine the next step.

If the second SUDS rating is 0, then you may be done with that "aspect or the issue." It is important to find a way to TEST the issue to be sure it really is gone, and that you haven't missed any aspects.

If the second SUDS rating is lower, then do another round of tapping, but this time change the Setup and Reminder Phrases to include, "This REMAINING..."

So the new Setup Phrase would be. "Even though I still have some of THIS REMAINING {problem statement} I deeply and completely love and accept myself."

You want to acknowledge that progress has been made, but also that there is still some of the issue remaining to be addressed with the next round of tapping.

<u>If SUDS rating has not changed</u> then look carefully to confirm that it really is the same issue, and you haven't moved on to the next tapping topic without realizing it. If you recognize that it's not the same issue, then consider it a new one, start again from the beginning, and address this new issue or aspect with a new round of tapping.

However, if it really is the same issue, then start over again and say the Setup Phrase out loud with EMPHASIS while tapping on the Karate Chop spot. Then tap through several rounds EFT before checking the SUDS again.

It is very unusual to have the second SUDS rating be higher than the first.

But if that is the case, then it is likely that either you have REALLY tuned into the issue much more effectively, or the more common situation is that you have shifted to another issue or aspect and have not recognized it.

Sometimes the shift can be subtle, so if you find yourself in this situation, I would suggest that you write down a COMPLETE description of the issue for comparison after the next round of tapping. Be sure to take notice of ANY differences in the Character, Location, or SUDS intensity when compared to the written description of the issue being addressed. I would also recommend doing several complete rounds of tapping, saying the Setup Phrase with EMPHASIS before checking the SUDS rating again

If you are really stuck, I would recommend being persistent. Try breaking the issue into smaller chunks. Be more specific in your problem description, and try working on it for several days in a row, doing several rounds of tapping each time.

If you are still really stuck I would suggest working with an EFT practitioner. Perhaps you are missing something that they will be able to see.

Summary of basic steps for EFT Tapping

- Choose an issue and create a "shorthand" description of it to use as the Reminder Phrase.
- Give it a SUDS rating.
- Do the Setup by tapping on the Karate Chop spot while saying out loud, three times: "Even though I have this {problem description} I deeply and completely love and accept myself."
- Then, while saying the Reminder Phrase out loud, do a couple of rounds of tapping through each of the points - EB, SE, UE, UN, CH, CB, UA, Top
- Finally, take a deep breath and give it a SUDS rating again.
- If there is still some SUDS intensity left, then do another complete round starting with the Setup Phrase and using "this remaining" along with the Reminder Phrase.

EFT Tapping Examples

Presented below are two of my favorite EFT Tapping teaching demonstrations. For most people they both are very effective at providing a personal experience of the type of shifts that using EFT Tapping can create with us.

If you happen to have access to some chocolate (or some other food that you can generate a high SUDS intensity of craving for it) then I would suggest that you try the craving demo first. And no, this exercise won't "make you hate chocolate" but it can demonstrate the power of EFT when it comes to creating a shift around cravings. And once you've personally experienced that kind of shift, it is much easier to have confidence in the EFT Tapping process and you are much more likely to apply it in other areas of your life too.

It should be noted that chocolate can be a Migraine symptom trigger for some people. So this demonstration could be particularly beneficial in reducing the craving for chocolate for those people. If chocolate is a Migraine trigger for you, you may want to consider modifying the demo, and not actually taste or eat the chocolate. This same craving demo could be used with other Migraine trigger foods as well. Simply replace the chocolate with your particular trigger food. And remember to always take responsibility for yourself and your wellbeing!

The second demo does a great job of demonstrating how "stress and tension" can affect our bodies and restrict our breathing – as measured with "perceived lung capacity" during this demonstration exercise. Even if you've participated in the craving demo I would still recommend participating in the second one. This is especially true if you want to address physical symptoms like Migraine Headaches through the use of EFT Tapping.

Craving Demo

When I do this teaching demonstration with a live audience, I usually have some Hershey's Kisses chocolate that we use as the "object of desire" so to speak. I like to use Kisses because they are small, come in bulk, and are individually wrapped, which makes them easier to hand out to each member of the class. They are also "just chocolate" rather than "really good chocolate" so there is less concern amongst the audience about "giving up their chocolate." If you happen to have some "just chocolate" available, then get it now, BUT DO NOT OPEN IT OR TAKE A BITE YET! And while you're getting it, grab a scrap of paper and a pen or pencil so you can write down your SUDS during the exercise.

Step 1) Intensify the desire (craving) for the chocolate!

Go ahead hold the chocolate in your hand and look at it while thinking about how good that chocolate will taste. Imagine unwrapping it, and the delicious smell of that chocolate first permeating your sense. Now imagine how good that chocolate would taste as it melts in your mouth. DO NOT take a bite yet, but do imagine it vividly.

Now write down on that scrap of paper how intensely you want that chocolate – Give it a "craving intensity" using the SUDS rating system you learned about earlier.

Now go ahead and actually unwrap a corner of the chocolate. Hold it up to your nose and get a good whiff of the smell of that delicious chocolate. Notice how the desire for that chocolate is making you feel right now. You may want to write a few words describing it and your current SUDS level.

Ok, it's time to take a little tiny bite of the chocolate – not a real bite, but just enough to get the flavor of the chocolate melting in your mouth without any hope of satisfying your desire to eat more of it.

Step 2) Write down the SUDS intensity of your desire or craving for that chocolate. Add a few words to describe how you are feeling about your desire to eat that chocolate!

Now put down the chocolate somewhere close where you can look at it during the rest of this demo sequence.

Step 3) While tapping continuously on the Karate Chop (KC) spot, say: "Even though I crave that chocolate, I deeply and completely love and accept myself. Even though I CRAVE that chocolate, I DEEPLY and COMPLETELY love and accept myself. Even though I crave that delicious, yummy chocolate, I deeply and completely love and accept myself."

Step 4) While looking at the chocolate, tap through each of the points while saying the Reminder Phrase "Crave That Chocolate!" at each point (to keep you focused on the craving itself.) Tap about 5-7 times on each location, or tap continuously for as long as it takes you to say the Reminder Phrase, "Crave That Chocolate!"

- Eyebrow (EB) – "Crave That Chocolate!"
- Side of the eye (SE) – "Crave That Chocolate!"
- Under the eye (UE) – "Crave That Chocolate!"
- Under the nose (UN) – "Crave That Chocolate!"
- Chin (CH) – "Crave That Chocolate!"
- Collar bone (CB) – "Crave That Chocolate!"
- Under the arm (UA) – "Crave That Chocolate!"
- Top of the head (Top) – "Crave That Chocolate!"

Do a second round of tapping exactly the same way – EB, SE, UE, UN, CH, CB, UA, Top – saying "Crave That Chocolate!" and tapping at each point.

Now take a deep breath, and release it.

Step 5) Check SUDS rating for the chocolate craving. Look at it for a moment and give the intensity of the craving for that chocolate a SUDS rating.

Now pick it up and smell it. Has the SUDS rating changed? How does this new SUDS rating compare with the one you wrote down before tapping? Is it lower? If so, by how much? (In rare cases it may have increased, which likely means that you've "tuned into" the craving even more!) Notice the feeling you have when you look at the chocolate and think about eating it. Has the feeling shifted or changed in any way when compared to what

EFT Tapping Examples

you wrote down? Go ahead, take another small taste, and see what you notice.

Write down this new SUDS rating again, along with any notes about the feelings you noticed.

Step 6) Another tapping round with "this remaining..."

While looking at the chocolate like you did during the first set of tapping, do another two rounds of tapping but change the Setup Phrase and the Reminder Phrase as shown below. The idea is to acknowledge that a shift has occurred AND that there is still a remaining SUDS intensity to focus on during this next group of tapping.

While looking at the chocolate and tapping continuously on the Karate Chop (KC) spot, say: "Even though I STILL crave that chocolate, I deeply and completely love and accept myself. Even though I STILL HAVE SOME OF THAT CHOCOLATE CRAVING, I DEEPLY and COMPLETELY love and accept myself. Even though I STILL HAVE SOME OF THIS REMAINING CRAVING for that delicious, yummy chocolate, I deeply and completely love and accept myself."

Continue to look at the chocolate while tapping through the points and saying "Remaining Chocolate Craving."

- Eyebrow – "Remaining Chocolate Craving"
- Side of the eye – "Remaining Chocolate Craving"
- Under the eye – "Remaining Chocolate Craving"
- Under the nose – "Remaining Chocolate Craving"
- Chin – "Remaining Chocolate Craving"
- Collar bone – "Remaining Chocolate Craving"
- Under the arm – "Remaining Chocolate Craving"

- Top of the head – "Remaining Chocolate Craving"

Do a second round of tapping exactly the same way – EB, SE, UE, UN, CH, CB, UA, Top – saying "Remaining Chocolate Craving" and tapping at each point.

Step 7) Again check your SUDS rating for the chocolate craving. Look at it for a moment and give the intensity of the craving for that chocolate a SUDS rating.

Now pick it up and smell it again. Has the SUDS rating changed? How does this new SUDS rating compare with the one you wrote down before tapping? Is it lower? If so, by how much? Notice the feeling you have when you look at the chocolate and think about eating it. Has the feeling shifted or changed in any way when compared to what you wrote down? Go ahead, take yet another small taste, and see what you notice.

Write down this new SUDS rating again, along with any notes about the feelings you noticed.

For most people who fully participate in this demonstration exercise there will be a noticeable shift in the SUDS intensity of the craving. There are often some bewildered looks in the room as they try to wrap their mind around the shift that they experienced "from this silly tapping thing" that they just did!

If you really want to have the full EFT Tapping experience, then go ahead and repeat steps 6 and 7 over again until your desire or craving for the chocolate drops to a SUDS rating of zero. I would encourage you to do a few more rounds of tapping, with the Setup, so that you can personally have the experience of getting to a SUDS of zero.

By the way, one of the things that is most unexpected for most people is the shift in the taste of the chocolate. For me, the first time that I did this with Hershey's Kisses, I noticed what I described as a "more chemical taste" than I had noticed originally.

As a quick aside here, Gary Craig also noticed something he calls "the apex effect" occurs sometimes. Occasionally people will go through a series of tapping on something that is bothering them emotionally, like a fear or traumatic memory, and at the end of the tapping, when their SUDS has dropped to zero, or close to zero, they will "wave off the results" of the tapping. Sometimes they'll say something like "the tapping distracted me from the problem," or "well, it wasn't really that much of a problem to begin with in the first place!" It's astonishing to watch. That is one of the reasons why I make sure when I am working with someone new to EFT Tapping that they write down, in their own handwriting, the SUDS rating at each step. It's harder to "deny the results" that way! And the idea isn't to beat them up about it, but to show them the results in black-and-white so they don't short-change themselves of the opportunity that EFT Tapping presents in their life.

As an enhancement to this book, I created a video showing the EFT Chocolate Craving Demo more clearly than can be done with words photos alone. You can see the video for the Chocolate Craving Demo here:

http://tapping4.us/chocolatedemo

You can find a complete list of videos and other internet content in the Resources section.

Breathing Demo

The EFT Tapping for Constricted Breathing demonstration is especially interesting in that it can clearly demonstrate the connection between EFT Tapping and the body's physical response. While this demo can be quite eye-opening for many people because of the degree of change that they notice, other people may only notice a small amount of shift. This demo works best in a group setting where a number of people can share their experiences with the exercise and the amount of shift they notice. It is well worth participating in this demo even if you are by yourself.

Another interesting aspect of this demo is that it will often "peel away layers of intensity" from general issues and allow you to remember specific events, or be able to describe the issue more clearly, so it can be addressed with further EFT Tapping.

This breathing demo includes bending over, so if you have Migraine symptoms now, you may want to come back to this demo later and try it after the Migraine symptoms are gone.

Step 1) "Stretch your lungs." The idea here is to take three really deep breaths in order to stretch your lungs a bit before establishing a baseline for the exercise. There is no need to hyperventilate, so take your time, and spread the deep breaths out over a couple of minutes.

One way to do this is to stand up, and exhale while you bend over forward and drop your arms toward the floor. Then inhale deeply as you stand up and raise your arms up and out so they are above your head. This will help to stretch and open your ribcage and allow for maximum expansion of your lungs.

EFT Tapping Examples

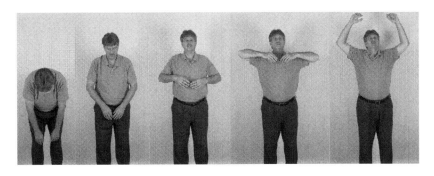

Step 2) Now that you have stretched your lungs as far as they will go, take another full deep breath and assess the "deepness of your breath" on a 0-10 scale, with 10 being your best estimate (or guess) of what your maximum lung capacity would be. Be sure to write it down on a scrap of paper for comparison later. Assigned values typically vary between 3 and 9 on this part of the exercise. (It is interesting to note that often the people who incorrectly assign a value of 10 for this beginning measurement, find that after several rounds of EFT Tapping they have to assign an ending value of 12 to 15 because of their assessment of the increase in lung capacity.)

Step 3) Next prepare to do several rounds of EFT Tapping by using a Setup Phrase like, "Even though I have constricted breathing..." or "Even though I can only fill my lungs to an 8..." for example.

Note: In the section below where I say "...fill my lungs to an 8..." substitute your number from Step 2 for the 8 in that phrase.

So, while tapping continuously on the Karate Chop (KC) spot, say: "Even though I have constricted breathing, I deeply and completely love and accept myself. Even though I have this constricted breathing, I DEEPLY and COMPLETELY love and accept myself. Even though I have constricted breathing and I can only fill my lungs to an 8, I deeply and completely love and accept myself."

Step 4) Now tap through each of the points while saying the Reminder Phrase "Constricted Breathing" at each point. Tap about five to seven times on each location, or tap continuously for as long as it takes you to say the Reminder Phrase.

- Eyebrow – "Constricted Breathing"
- Side of the eye – "Constricted Breathing"
- Under the eye – "Constricted Breathing"
- Under the nose – "Constricted Breathing"
- Chin – "Constricted Breathing"
- Collar bone – "Constricted Breathing"
- Under the arm – "Constricted Breathing"
- Top of the head – "Constricted Breathing"

After you have completed this round of tapping, take another full deep breath, the same way you did before tapping, and assess the "deepness of your breath" on a 0-10 scale, then write it down and compare it to your original assessment.

Next, do a second round of tapping exactly the same way – EB, SE, UE, UN, CH, CB, UA, Top – while saying "I can only fill my lungs to an 8" as you are tapping at each point.

- Eyebrow – "I can only fill my lungs to an 8"
- Side of the eye – "I can only fill my lungs to an 8"
- Under the eye – "I can only fill my lungs to an 8"
- Under the nose – "I can only fill my lungs to an 8"
- Chin – "I can only fill my lungs to an 8"

- Collar bone – "I can only fill my lungs to an 8"
- Under the arm – "I can only fill my lungs to an 8"
- Top of the head – "I can only fill my lungs to an 8"

After you have completed this second round of tapping, take another full deep breath and assess the "deepness of your breath" on a 0-10 scale, then write it down and compare it to your original assessment.

Next, do a third round of tapping exactly the same way – EB, SE, UE, UN, CH, CB, UA, Top – while alternating between saying "Constricted Breathing" and "I can only fill my lungs to an 8" as you are tapping at each point. (Alternating what you are saying helps to keep you focused and engaged and alleviates some of the boredom that comes with always saying the same thing.)

- Eyebrow – "Constricted Breathing"
- Side of the eye – "I can only fill my lungs to an 8"
- Under the eye – "Constricted Breathing"
- Under the nose – "I can only fill my lungs to an 8"
- Chin – "Constricted Breathing"
- Collar bone – "I can only fill my lungs to an 8"
- Under the arm – "Constricted Breathing"
- Top of the head – "I can only fill my lungs to an 8"

After you have completed this third round of tapping, take yet another full deep breath, the same way you did before tapping, and assess the "deepness of your breath" on a 0-10 scale, then write it down and compare it to your original and second round assessments.

Most people will be a bit shocked to find that their perceived lung capacity has increased during this demonstration. Some people will even have "interesting answers" to questions like, "What does this constricted breathing remind you of?" "When in your past did your feel constricted or smothered?" "If there was an emotional reason for this constricted breathing, what might it be?" Often these will lead to fruitful areas for exploration and further EFT Tapping. It is often very useful to make note of those memories, ideas, and insights that present themselves in these situations. They can often lead to big clues about important emotional issues than can be further addressed using EFT Tapping.

Online video example

While the internet is ever changing, at the time of publication of this book you can find a video of a group "constricted breathing" demonstration on Gary Craig's website through this link:

http://tapping4.us/breathing

Troubleshooting Tips For Common Difficulties In Applying EFT Tapping

EFT Tapping can be applied to a wide variety of things in your life. Listed below are some common difficulties and suggestions for how to resolve them.

Being too general

One of the most common causes of difficulty in creating results with EFT Tapping is being too general with the issue definition. Go for the SPECIFIC FEELING and where it is located in your body, especially when dealing with physical issues.

Or you could address a specific EVENT (or memory of an event) that is bothering you. Don't lump things together into a group of similar items. Separate them out and address them each individually.

Losing track of the issue

One of the challenges with EFT Tapping is that things shift so quickly sometimes that you lose track of exactly what the problem was. I recommend writing down the exact description of what you are addressing with each round of tapping. It helps you stay focused on the exact issue and helps you to spot the subtle changes that sometimes occur. This is particularly true with physical issues, and helps you to recognize when things are shifting as you "chase the pain." Sometimes it appears that the SUDS intensity is the same, but upon closer inspection you will notice that the Character has changed – from sharp pain to dull ache, for example. This does represent a shift and should be considered as progress toward resolution as well.

Say it like it is so you can address the actual issue

Also don't "sugar coat it," or minimize it, or be politically correct with the definition of the issue. Say how you really feel and use YOUR actual phrasing! Don't say, "I don't like to exercise," when you really feel that, "Exercise is a pain in the ass!"

You are trying to TUNE INTO the ACTUAL issue so you can address it and release it! But you can't tune into it if you're not saying it "like it is" and in a way that matches your actual feelings!

Skipping steps

Another common cause of difficulties is skipping steps. If you are not tapping on the Karate Chop spot (KC) and using the Setup Phrase, and you're making slow progress or no progress, then go back, add in the Setup Phrase, and say it with EMPHASIS while tapping on the KC. And remember to be specific with the description of the issue!

Addressing an undefined or poorly specified issue

Another difficulty that may show up is struggling with defining the issue or not finding something specific on which to tap. Remember that you can always tap on the Feeling in your body that comes up when you think about an issue.

You could also tap on "Even though I don't know why I'm feeling this way..." or "Even though I can't clearly define the issue..." or something like that.

Fast Migraine Headache Relief With EFT Tapping

EFT Tapping on a Page

Emotional Freedom Technique – Summary Overview

Choose an issue to work on and Rate **SUDS intensity**

SETUP: **Tap** continuously on **KC** while **saying Setup Phrase 3 times**:

"**Even though {problem statement} I deeply and completely love and accept myself.**"

While saying **reminder phrase** (the "short version" of the problem statement) **tap** about 7 times on each spot while tapping through the sequence:

EB, SE, UE, UN CH, CB, UA, Top

Do **2 or more rounds** of tapping through the sequence and **then check SUDS** again

If **SUDS = 0**, you are probably done with that aspect. **TEST** to be sure!

If **SUDS has decreased** do another round of tapping with "...REMAINING..."

- SETUP: Even though <u>I still have some of THIS REMAINING</u> {problem statement} I deeply and completely love and accept myself.
- Reminder Phrase:
  THIS REMAINING {short version of problem statement}
- Do 2 or more rounds of tapping through the sequence and then check SUDS again

If **SUDS has increased**: Is it REALLY the same issue?

- Yes: tap on KC & say SETUP OUT LOUD WITH EMPHASIS! Then tap 3 or more rounds while focusing on issue
- No: It' a new aspect or issue
  – Start from the beginning again.

Focus on the feeling while saying reminder phrase & tapping!

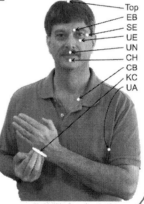

© 2013 Transformation Bay LLC

Download and print out your full color, full size copy here:

http://tapping4.us/cheat-sheet

Section 2: Applying EFT Tapping For Fast Migraine Headache Relief

DISCLAIMER: The content presented here is for informational purposes only. It is not medical advice and should not be taken as medical advice. You are advised to check with a qualified medical practitioner before taking any action based on this information. See the disclaimer at the beginning of this book for more information.

How to use this section

This section dives into the details on how to apply EFT Tapping specifically for Migraine Headache symptoms.

If a Migraine Headache is starting now...

...then I would recommend that you immediately turn to the "Migraine Tapping Fast Start" section and simply follow along while doing what is shown there.

If you don't have Migraine symptoms right now...

...then I would suggest reading through this material and following along with the exercises so that you are familiar with how to apply EFT Tapping for a Migraine Headache before the next one starts.

Getting Started With Migraine Headache EFT Tapping

In many ways EFT Tapping for Migraine Headache symptoms is exactly like addressing any other physical symptom with EFT Tapping. The idea is that you focus on the symptoms and tap. The process is guided through the symptom reduction process toward completion by noting the SUDS intensity, Character, and Location of the symptoms, while "chasing the pain" as it is often described.

Using SUDS, Character, and Location to guide your tapping process

As defined earlier in this book SUDS stands for Subject Units of Distress Scale and the arbitrary 0-10 scale that is used to "measure" the intensity of the symptoms. Zero is assigned to no intensity, while 10 is assigned to "being as intense as you can imagine it to be." By using the SUDS to assess the intensity before and after rounds of tapping, you are able to more easily notice and quantify the shifts that are occurring.

The "Character of a symptom" may include descriptors like Sharp, Dull, Throbbing, Stabbing, Achy, Nausea, Dizziness, or any other descriptive word that applies. It's not the exact Character that is important, but rather the change in Character that influences the process. Feel free to choose whatever words describe the "Character" of the symptom for you, but be sure that you know exactly what that definition is for you so that you can notice the shift.

Location may be one of the easiest factors to quantify. It is often the case that one is able to note the "exact" Location of a symptom or pain on the physical body – "behind and slightly above my left eye socket," for example. Again it is not the exact Location that matters but the shift in what you are noticing that guides the process.

I will often recommend to people who are just starting out using EFT Tapping that they write down the SUDS, Character, and Location information so that they are 100% certain of the description of their "starting conditions." This information is especially helpful when they come back to assess the change after the first and subsequent rounds of tapping. It removes any uncertainty and helps build confidence in the process and experience.

Example Tapping Script Walk-Through

The following is an example tapping script walk-through that shows the whole process, including the decision points and the criteria that are used to make the choices on how to proceed. It is an abbreviated version of what you may experience in that you may need to do several more rounds of tapping than are described here. However, by following this example it should be clear to you exactly what to do, and how to make your choices on how to proceed through the process based on the SUDS, Character, and Location for your particular situation and symptoms.

For this example we will assume that it is the middle of the afternoon and you notice that you have the beginning of a Migraine Headache. You've been very busy since lunch and intensely focused on several different tasks that were taking your full attention so you didn't notice the early pre-cursor symptoms.

SUDS, Character, & Location – Initial Assessment

You have just had a momentary break in your intense focus and have noticed the following symptoms:

A dull and throbbing pain slightly behind and above the inside edge of your left eye with a SUDS intensity rating of a 5. Tension in the muscles of your scalp, with a general SUDS intensity of a 3, but it is stronger on the left side above your ear with a SUDS of 4 in that area. Your vision is slightly "off" but full-blown auras haven't started yet so it has a SUDS of 2.

Notice that there are three distinct symptom descriptions here – The pain, the tension, and the vision symptoms. The highest SUDS rating is a 5 for the pain, so that is the issue to focus on initially.

Setup Phrase and KC tapping

The description above for the SUDS, Character, and Location is quite long, so it would be impractical to repeat it every time as the Setup Phrase and Reminder Phrase. As a result, you could create a shorthand version of it. Since we are going to focus on the pain for the initial tapping rounds we will use the short-had description, "This 5 throbbing eye pain" to represent the longer and more complete description.

Now you can start the EFT Tapping process by tapping continuously on the KC or "karate chop" spot, (see diagram) while repeating the Setup Phrase, three times, "Even though I have this 5 throbbing eye pain, I deeply and completely love and accept myself."

Tapping through the points

Next you would tap through each of the locations while repeating the Reminder Phrase "This 5 throbbing eye pain." (Tap about five to seven times on each location, or tap continuously for as long as it takes you to say the Reminder Phrase.)

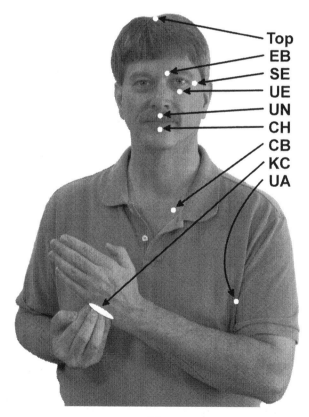

- Eyebrow – "This 5 throbbing eye pain."
- Side of the eye – "This 5 throbbing eye pain."
- Under the eye – "This 5 throbbing eye pain."
- Under the nose – "This 5 throbbing eye pain."
- Chin – "This 5 throbbing eye pain."
- Collar bone – "This 5 throbbing eye pain."
- Under the arm – "This 5 throbbing eye pain."
- Top of the head – "This 5 throbbing eye pain."

Then do a second round of tapping exactly the same way – EB, SE, UE, UN, CH, CB, UA, Top – saying "This 5 throbbing eye pain" and tapping at each point.

Now take a deep breath, and release it.

SUDS, Character, & Location reassessment

It is now time to reassess the SUDS, Character, and Location of the symptoms. At this point we will assume that the long description represented by "This 5 throbbing eye pain" has not changed, but the intensity has reduced from a SUDS rating of a 5 to a 3.

It shifted

Because the long description of the symptom has remained the same but the SUDS intensity has dropped, we would do another round of EFT Tapping with the updated Reminder Phrase "This REMAINING throbbing eye pain." In this case we want to acknowledge that the SUDS intensity has shifted lower but there is still some remaining pain to be addressed.

Tapping through the points – Round 2

For the next round of tapping we will take a calculated risk and skip the Setup-KC Tapping segment, since it is only needed about 40% of the time, and we also used it before the first round of tapping (which I always recommend!)

Tapping through the points...

- Eyebrow – "This remaining throbbing eye pain."
- Side of the eye – "This remaining throbbing eye pain."
- Under the eye – "This remaining throbbing eye pain."
- Under the nose – "This remaining throbbing eye pain."
- Chin – "This remaining throbbing eye pain."
- Collar bone – "This remaining throbbing eye pain."
- Under the arm – "This remaining throbbing eye pain."
- Top of the head – "This remaining throbbing eye pain."

Then do a second round of tapping exactly the same way – EB, SE, UE, UN, CH, CB, UA, Top – saying "This remaining throbbing eye pain" and tapping at each point.

Now take a deep breath, and release it.

SUDS, Character, & Location reassessment after round 2

It is now time to again reassess the SUDS, Character, and Location of the symptoms. At this point you may do a quick check in and notice that the SUDS intensity is still a 3.

It didn't change - so what happened?

This is an area where people will often get confused. The last paragraph wasn't explicit in what was being measured just that the SUDS intensity was still a 3. Many people stumble over this in real life. They will note the overall SUDS intensity of the "most intense symptom" but not notice that it isn't the same symptom as was addressed in the last tapping round.

One way to help prevent this from happening is to write down the details for the symptom that you are tapping on for a particular round of tapping. That way you can check back in and see exactly where you started and what you were focused on for that round of tapping.

For the sake of this example, we will assume that the "throbbing eye pain" SUDS intensity has dropped to a 0, 1, or 2 which makes the "scalp muscle tension" the most intense symptom at a 3 which is overshadowing the "throbbing eye pain" so it isn't noticed.

So for this next round of tapping we will assume that the "throbbing eye pain" is no longer obvious since it is "hiding behind" the "scalp muscle tension." The eye pain may continue to shift lower as you tap on other symptoms. If not, then as the intensity of the other symptoms subside it may resurface for further tapping attention.

Tapping through the points – Round 3

Since we are now dealing with a different symptom than in the last tapping round, we will again start with the Setup and KC tapping. Tap continuously on the KC while repeating the Setup Phrase, three times, "Even though I have this scalp muscle tension, I deeply and completely love and accept myself."

Now tapping through the points...

- Eyebrow – "This scalp muscle tension."
- Side of the eye – "This scalp muscle tension."
- Under the eye – "This scalp muscle tension."
- Under the nose – "This scalp muscle tension."
- Chin – "This scalp muscle tension."
- Collar bone – "This scalp muscle tension."
- Under the arm – "This scalp muscle tension."
- Top of the head – "This scalp muscle tension."

Then do a second round of tapping exactly the same way – EB, SE, UE, UN, CH, CB, UA, Top – saying "This remaining scalp muscle tension" and tapping at each point.

Now take a deep breath, and release it.

SUDS, Character, & Location reassessment after round 3

It is now time to again reassess the SUDS, Character, and Location of the symptoms. At this point, you may notice that each of the symptoms has substantially subsided in SUDS intensity. While each and every symptom may not have fallen to a zero, you could choose to call it complete here. I would, however, encourage you to continue the EFT tapping process and apply it to every symptom until each one is as close to zero as is reasonably practical. Sometime SUDS levels of 1 or below will finish dissipating over time, but why risk it when another couple of minutes of tapping may finish it off.

As an enhancement to this book, I created a video showing the Migraine EFT Tapping Script Walk Through more clearly than can be done with words photos alone. You can see the Migraine EFT Tapping Script Walk Through video here:

http://tapping4.us/migrainewalkthru.

You can find a complete list of videos and other internet content in the Resources section.

Important things to watch for...

...especially if your progress is slow

Focus on the feeling

One of the keys to tapping success is to focus on the feelings and sensations. It is often easier to simply notice and assess what is going on than to really stop and think about it in order to analyze the details. The whole point of assessing the SUDS, Character, and Location is to create a frame of reference with which to notice and measure the shifts that are taking place.

Add Setup Phrase

Sometimes I will choose not to do the Setup and KC tapping before each set of tapping rounds. That is a calculated risk that comes with experience. The key thing to remember is that if you are "not making progress" as defined by the SUDS reducing, then go ahead and add the Setup and KC tapping back in, and be sure to say the Setup Phrase with emphasis! It is amazing how much of a difference that will make sometimes.

This concludes the Example Tapping Script Walk-Through.

Fast Migraine Headache Relief With EFT Tapping

EFT On A Page Cheat Sheet Migraine Edition

EFT On A Page Cheat Sheet – Migraine Edition

Reminder: Start EFT Tapping at first sign of symptoms.

Assess & note: SUDS, Character, Location of symptoms & create *shorthand description* for use while tapping.

Setup: Tap KC continuously while saying setup phrase 3x

"Even though {symptom description} I deeply and completely love and accept myself."

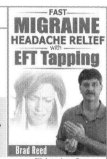
Click to buy On Amazon.com

While saying *shorthand description* reminder phrase tap about 7x on each spot while tapping through the sequence:

EB, SE, UE, UN, CH, CB, UA, Top.

Do 2+ rounds of tapping through the sequence, then reassess.

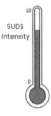

If Character & Location are the same but SUDS decreased: do another round of taping with "this remaining"

- Setup 3x: "Even though I <u>still have some of this remaining</u> {symptom description} I deeply and completely love and Accept myself."
- Reminder Phrase: <u>This remaining</u> {shorthand description}
- Do 2 or more rounds of tapping through the sequence & reassess.

If Character or Location changed, start again with Setup & new SUDS, Character, Location description. Tap through again.

"Chase the pain" - Reassess & tap again on new SUDS, Character, & Location.

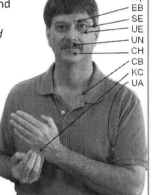

Visit http://WithEFTtapping.com/book-migraine **for more**

Download and print out your full color, full size copy here:

http://tapping4.us/migraine-book-cheat-sheet

Migraine Tapping Fast Start

This section assumes that you are taking complete personal responsibility for yourself and your wellbeing, and that you have checked with a qualified medical practitioner before starting to apply the EFT Tapping methods described here.

If you have read the prior sections of this book, including the disclaimer, and participated in the demo exercises, then you have a good understanding of what is going to be presented here and the thinking behind it.

If this is the first section of this book that you are reading, please go back and read the Disclaimer page before proceeding. The bottom line is that you must take personal responsibility for yourself and your own health and wellbeing and it is assumed that you have checked with a qualified health practitioner before participating in the EFT Tapping described below. If that is not the case, then proceed no further until you have done so.

Step 1) Note the Location, Character, and SUDS intensity of your Migraine Headache symptoms. (Example: A dull and throbbing pain slightly behind and

Fast Migraine Headache Relief With EFT Tapping

above the inside edge of your left eye with an intensity rating of a 5 on the SUDS 0-10 scale.)

Step 2) While tapping on the (KC) Karate Chop spot (see diagram below) say out loud, "Even though I have these Migraine Headache symptoms, I deeply and completely love and accept myself," and at the point where you say "these Migraine Headache symptoms" pause for a moment while focusing on the specific Location, Character, and SUDS intensity of the symptoms. The idea is to be very clear about what you are intending to shift by "looking at" the way it is right now.

Do this KC Tapping step three times.

Step 3) Tap through each of the points shown in the diagram while repeating the Reminder Phrase "these Migraine Headache symptoms." (Tap about five to seven times on each location, or tap continuously for as long as it takes you to say the Reminder Phrase.)

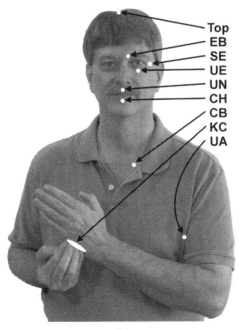

- Eyebrow – "These Migraine Headache symptoms."
- Side of the eye – "These Migraine Headache symptoms."
- Under the eye – "These Migraine Headache symptoms."
- Under the nose – "These Migraine Headache symptoms."
- Chin – "These Migraine Headache symptoms."
- Collar bone – "These Migraine Headache symptoms."
- Under the arm – "These Migraine Headache symptoms."
- Top of the head – "These Migraine Headache symptoms."

Then do a second round of tapping exactly the same way – EB, SE, UE, UN, CH, CB, UA, Top – saying "These Migraine Headache symptoms" and tapping at each point.

Now take a deep breath, and release it.

Step 4) Reassess the Location, Character, and SUDS intensity of your Migraine Headache symptoms and compare them to your first assessment.

If the Location and Character are EXACTLY the same, but the SUDS intensity has shifted lower, then do another few rounds of EFT Tapping but replace the Reminder Phrase with "These REMAINING Migraine Headache symptoms." Then revisit Step 4 to determine what to do next.

If the Location and/or the Character has changed, then go back to Step 1 and treat this as a "new" version of the Migraine symptoms. The idea here is that you are "chasing the pain" and doing a few rounds of tapping on each "version" of the pain in order to reduce the SUDS intensity. In this case since you noticed a shift in Location and/or Character, it is considered a "new version" of the symptoms and you start at the beginning with Step 1. This should be seen as progress because the "old version" of the symptoms have been released (or at least are no longer as prominent as the "new version").

Continue to "chase the symptoms" by doing several rounds of EFT Tapping for each "new set of symptoms" as defined by changes in the Location and/or Character of the symptoms. When you notice it is just the SUDS intensity that has changed, simply tap through the points again using "this remaining..." in addition to the original Reminder Phrase.

Eventually, after several rounds of tapping, you are likely to find that the Migraine Headache symptoms have either A) substantially subsided, or B) not changed much, in which case you need to remember that you have agreed to take complete personal responsibility for yourself and your wellbeing, and it may be time to consider other treatment options for moving toward Migraine symptom relief.

If your symptoms have substantially subsided but are not "completely gone" then I would recommend a few more rounds of EFT Tapping using the "chase the symptom" technique until they are pretty much gone. You should also remember that if the symptoms start to come back you can do the same sort of tapping procedure for those symptoms as well.

The first time I helped a friend of mine with her Migraine, she got fast initial relief using EFT Tapping, but she did have to do additional tapping both times the symptoms started to reoccur that same day. She started tapping as soon as she noticed the symptoms and did not wait for their SUDS intensity to climb. I would recommend the same strategy for you.

As an enhancement to this book, I created a video showing the Migraine Tapping Fast Start more clearly than can be done with words photos alone. You can see the Migraine Tapping Fast Start video here:

http://tapping4.us/migrainefaststart

You can find a complete list of videos and other internet content in the Resources section.

This concludes the "Migraine Tapping Fast Start" section.

Using EFT Tapping To Address Migraine Triggers

One of Gary Craig's biggest points in his teaching is the link between emotions and physical symptoms. One doesn't have to look very far to see examples of that link operating in each of our own lives. So it probably doesn't seem like much of a stretch to consider the idea that emotions may be one of the contributing factors that could trigger Migraine symptoms. And the first step to changing that situation is to raise one's awareness of possible triggers and recognize those that do show up in our lives.

Recognizing triggers

For simplicity's sake, let's break the pool of potential Migraine triggers into two sections – physical triggers and emotional triggers. It should be noted that there are a variety of causes for Migraine symptoms. It could be a food or environmental sensitivity, a nutritional deficiency, a hormonal imbalance, or even something more serious like a tumor. As always, it is important to take responsibility for yourself and consult with a licensed health care provider.

Physical Triggers

Physical triggers could be things like food or environmental factors. Your doctor is likely to suggest a list of potential triggers that may include things like food preservatives (e.g., nitrates, MSG), alcohol and red wine, coffee, tea, and cola, artificial sweeteners, and even specific foods like aged cheeses, chocolate, citrus fruits, nuts and peanut butter, or even salty foods. Environmental factors might include smoke or smog, chemical odors, perfumes and fragrances, weather, and temperature or barometric pressure changes.

Some of these factors are obviously beyond our control, like the weather, while others may be within our control, like food choices. In either case, there is likely to be a benefit that comes from being aware of what may trigger Migraine symptoms for you.

It may seem rather odd to suggest trying this, but there are cases where people have applied EFT Tapping with the intention to shift food, or environmental, sensitivities and have noticed positive results.

I know that I have personally used EFT Tapping to create shifts in unexpected areas. There was a time about a decade ago where I was fairly lactose intolerant, and it showed up as stomach upset. I was personally able to apply EFT Tapping, over time and with creatively focusing on a number of possible aspects, and I significantly reduced my "apparent lactose intolerance." While I can't guarantee that sort of result for you, I hope that I have intrigued you enough to consider looking into how to apply EFT Tapping to that sort of thing in your life.

My point in sharing that story with you is that our bodies are amazingly intelligent organic machines and they can shift and change in potentially unexpected ways based on our physical and "emotional environment."

Emotional triggers

Emotional triggers for Migraine symptoms may not be as obvious, when first considered, as environmental triggers can be. However if we consider the wide variety of ways that our body may respond to stress, it becomes more obvious

Stress

Stress can be a contributing factor as a Migraine trigger in a number of ways. The medical community has recognized that not only can high levels of stress trigger Migraines, but it is sometimes the cumulative effect of stress that can trigger them as well. On the opposite end there is also evidence that stress letdown on weekends, vacations, or even after the ending of a stressful project can act as a trigger.

EFT Tapping can be used, especially on a regular basis, to reduce your overall stress level, thus reducing the likelihood of Migraine symptoms. You could start by tapping on "...all this stress..." which is fairly broad, and then after a few rounds of tapping on that, dig in deeper and focus on more specific things like, "...my boss is riding me to get this done...", "...I can't believe I have to bail them out and fix this again!" or even "...I can't believe they are such idiots! Can't they see what the real problem is?" Simply choose the wording that describes the focus of your stress and start tapping!

Many times simply giving voice to the stressful thoughts that are running through your head WHILE TAPPING CONTINUOUSLY and speaking them will really take the edge off your stress level. If you are like most humans today, you probably have a natural propensity to want to "bitch and complain" about the things that are upsetting to you or bothering you. The good news is that by actually voicing those thoughts out loud while tapping you are very likely to notice a shift in the intensity level of those feelings. It may take more than a few minutes, especially if there are a lot of them, but in the end when I do that, I find my stress level greatly reduced at least for a while. Because I know this is such a powerful strategy, I even created a website that focuses on this method. You can find it at

http://www.TapAndBitch.com

When you enter your name and email address in the box in the upper right-hand corner of the site, you will be sent access to a free 23-minute video that I created called The EFT Quick Start Video Learning System. I would strongly recommend that you check it out. (Not to be crude or offense, but "TapAndComplain.com" simply doesn't have the same impact and isn't nearly as memorable either.)

A quick side note here for those who follow The Law Of Attraction so they are disinclined to want to focus on "negative things," but rather try to keep their outlook and attitude positive. As the author of The Secret For Law Of Attraction video training program, which is available through Amazon.com, I can definitely tell you that if you "focus on the negative" for long enough to apply EFT Tapping and "release the energy you have around it" you will be FAR more successful with the Law Of Attraction! That is because you are likely to find that the thoughts and feelings that you have tapped on simply don't show up as often. Through tapping you have "taken the emotional charge off" those things and as a result you naturally spend less time thinking about them and thus less time reminding yourself to "not think about them or put your attention there," because they simply don't come up! Consider these two scenarios: On one hand you could spend 10-15 minutes actually "focusing on the negative thing" while you are tapping on it so that it is released which can result in those thoughts "visiting" you less, and having lower intensity. On the other hand you could spend a minute each day "accidentally" thinking about the negative until you catch yourself and focus elsewhere on something more positive. How many minutes do you think you would accumulate in a month for each scenario? I'm willing to put my money on the tapping route.

Give it a try, and I think you'll be pleasantly surprised.

Anticipation induced stress

Sometimes we can work ourselves up into quite a stress-filled state when we are anticipating a future event that we expect to be challenging. This sort of thing can really create a peak in stress and thus potentially trigger Migraine symptoms.

Applying EFT Tapping to what you are afraid MIGHT happen, (since it hasn't occurred yet, you really don't know if it even will) can often be a way to not only lower your stress level but get into a more resourceful state where you can better plan and respond to what happens rather than simply reacting from your fears.

You could tap on things like "...I don't know what's going to happen..." or "...I'm afraid that (fill-in-the-blank) will happen..." or "...I don't know what I will do if (fill-in-the-blank) happens..." etc. Voicing it while tapping through the points will likely reduce your stress level at that moment.

The flip side of this could also be a Migraine symptom trigger. It doesn't have to be "negative stress." It could be the stress of extreme anticipation of something good too. The body may not be able to distinguish between the two, so tapping would probably be beneficial for both situations.

People, Anger, Power & Control

Without getting too deep into this, let me just say that it would not be unheard of for people in your life to "trigger Migraine symptoms." If we were to dig into this deeper I could probably build a decent case for the idea that Migraine symptoms could be your body's extreme way of trying to "protect itself" while keeping you safe and out of an otherwise "bad" situation.

Take this scenario for example. Let's just say that hypothetically, you and your mother-in-law don't get along well...at all! And let's just say that every time you visit with her, or are in her presence, things "go badly" to put it mildly. So every time you even get a hint that you may be around her soon your stress level goes way up. And as the scheduled event draws nearer, your stress level continues to climb. In this sort of situation, you may find that Migraine symptoms start to show up right before it is time to leave for the event, thus preventing you from attending. If you find that this cycle is happening repeatedly, it may be possible that your body's intelligence has "found a way to keep you safe" by preventing the interaction with your mother-in-law at that event. Obviously this is an extreme example, but it illustrates the point.

Now consider shifting the scenario so that the primary emotion is anger. The more intense the anger, the higher the stress level. And a similar mechanism may show up.

The reason I'm sharing these stories is to provide you with an opportunity to see things through a different lens. There may be (and often is!) more going on under the surface than meets the eye. Tapping is a wonderful tool to help you address many situations in your life and reduce your overall stress level as well. But in order to take your tapping skills to the next level where you have even more leverage and can shift things with deeper root causes, you need to develop some "detective skills" to help uncover those deeper issues.

Throughout this book, I have endeavored to share with you many of my "tricks of the trade" and secrets that I use to get faster and deeper results with EFT Tapping both for my clients and myself.

Tapping for triggers

In previous sections I've made various suggestions about how to approach issues and some options for specific wording. They represent a good "jumping off point" to start your journey into tapping for triggers. One of the key things to remember is to keep tapping and exploring any possible options for "things to tap on" that could lead to relief. Persistence will be your best friend in this case. It may take some time, and some digging, to find the origins of the issue so you can release it at its roots.

In addition to the ideas and suggestions included in this book, additional resources that can assist you in this journey can be found in the resource section toward the back of this book.

The power of persistence

Sometimes things just don't go right or work out the way you expect them to. This can be the case for EFT Tapping too, just like anything else. In general, the "worst" that will happen is you may waste a little bit of time doing some tapping on an issue, or symptom, and it doesn't seem to want to budge after 3-4 rounds of your best tapping technique. If you find that to be the case, I would suggest a couple of things. (As was stated before, first and foremost you need to take responsibility for your own wellbeing and do what you think is right for your situation.)

My first suggestion would be come back and try again later. Sometimes that's all it will take, simply a fresh approach on a different day. Another suggestion would be to enlist the help of a "tapping buddy" who is "outside" of the problem or issue and may be able to give you a fresh perspective and point out something you overlooked or otherwise missed. I know that's been the case for me sometimes.

The point is to continue to persist in applying EFT Tapping in your life. As is pointed out in other sections of this book, EFT tapping can be applied to a wide variety of situations and symptoms, and many, many people get great results by using it in their life. Persistence in applying it in your life will very likely lead to a similar result.

Tapping Frequently Asked Questions

In anticipation that people will skip around within this section, I have included the "check with a qualified medical practitioner" comment in several of the answers. There is some additional repetition of comments within this section so that each of the answers can stand by itself and be complete.

Do I need to check with my Doctor before I start using EFT Tapping?

As with anything health related, you should always check with a qualified medical practitioner before starting any new program. That applies to EFT Tapping as well. While there is growing study-based evidence that has been published in scholarly peer review journals, the traditional medical community has not yet "officially endorsed" the use of EFT Tapping. One published example is Dr. David Feinstein's article <u>Acupoint Stimulation in Treating Psychological Disorders: Evidence of Efficacy</u> that was published in 2012 in

Review of General Psychology (Vol 16(4), Dec 2012, 364-380) which is a flagship journal of the American Psychological Association. You can read more about it here:

http://tapping4.us/research-feinstein.

For more links to scholarly studies see the Resources section at the back of this book.

Who can use EFT Tapping?

Pretty much anyone can use EFT Tapping to help alleviate their Migraine Headache symptoms. You can even help someone else by doing the verbalization and tapping for them. However, as with anything health related, you should always check with a qualified medical practitioner before starting any new program, including applying EFT.

Is it safe for kids to use EFT Tapping?

Pretty much anyone can use EFT Tapping, including kids, to help alleviate their Migraine Headache symptoms. You can even help a child who is too young to do the tapping themselves by doing the verbalization and tapping for them. However, as with anything health related, you should always check with a qualified medical practitioner before starting any new program.

Is it safe to use EFT Tapping for other things?

Within the normal parameters of anything health related - you should always check with a qualified medical practitioner before starting any new program – I'd give it a great big "yes!" I've personally used EFT Tapping to deal with or alleviate symptoms of a wide variety of things. I've helped people get over their Fear of

Flying, Fear of Heights, Migraine Headaches and much, much, more. Gary Craig, the creator of EFT has said for years, "Try it on everything!" And I would echo that sentiment.

Which side do I tap on – Right or Left?

The general consensus is that it really doesn't matter which side you tap on. I generally tap on both sides, and I tap with two fingers so I cover a larger area while I'm tapping. That way I don't have to worry about hitting the exact tapping location and I can concentrate on focusing on the issue at hand instead.

How hard do I tap?

I generally tap with two fingers about as hard as I would press on a computer keyboard when I am typing. I use two fingers so that I am covering a slightly larger tapping area and can focus on the tapping and the Reminder Phrase, instead of wondering if I'm getting the exact tapping location.

When should I start tapping?

For Migraine Headaches, I'd start tapping at the very first sign that one is starting. Many people will notice a set of feelings or sensations that are often a precursor to a Migraine Headache. Personally, that's when I'd start tapping on those specific symptoms as well as my "fear that I'm about to get a Migraine Headache."

Personally, I start tapping anytime I notice something that I want to shift. I'd even suggest doing some tapping while you are walking to get your normal Migraine Headache medicine or treatment. It's likely you've got a few moments between when you notice the Migraine starting and when you take action to start your normal treatment protocol, so try tapping then (if you even wait THAT long!)

How long should I tap?

This question is somewhat tricky to answer. On the first level, I would say tap until the symptoms are gone. However, you need to take responsibility for yourself and your health and wellbeing. (As with anything health related, you should always check with a qualified medical practitioner before starting any new program.) So perhaps a better answer is that I would encourage you to at least invest a few minutes tapping before taking other measures to get relief. If EFT Tapping is working for you and getting you some relief, then I'd continue tapping and focusing on all the various ways I could think of to approach the problem, until I had achieved my goal of symptom relief. On the other hand, if I wasn't noticing any significant shift after a few rounds of tapping (maybe 3-4 rounds) then I would move on to other options for symptom relief. And I would still try EFT Tapping next time at the first sign of Migraine symptoms.

How often should I tap?

I would apply EFT Tapping any (and every) time that I noticed symptoms of a Migraine Headache. And if the symptoms dissipated and then started to return, I'd start tapping again. The very first woman I taught how to apply EFT Tapping to a Migraine, noticed symptom relief in a few minutes. However, she also noticed that over the next few hours the symptoms starting to return, so she applied EFT Tapping again both times and was Migraine free for the rest of the day. Now I can't guarantee that will be your experience, but the point is that she did the "right thing" and tapped again when the symptoms started to return. And she was rewarded by successfully preventing it from developing into something more severe. (As with anything health related, you should always check with a qualified medical practitioner before starting any new program.)

How do I know that it's working?

There are a number ways that you can notice that EFT Tapping is having the desired result. First, you are likely to notice that your SUDS rating is shifting lower, and that's a great sign that you're making progress. Second, you may notice that you are yawning (or even burping!) in the middle of tapping. I've personally noticed that this will often occur for me and is a personal indicator that "shift is happening." Third, you may notice a sigh, or other release of general body tension. Fourth, you may notice a shift in your viewpoint, attitude, or outlook about the issue. Things that used to be very "big" for you simply aren't much of an issue for you anymore. And finally, you may simply "notice a shift" and that's the only way you can describe it.

What should I do when I notice a shift?

The short answer is keep tapping if your SUDS isn't zero yet! However, there are two primary things to consider that fall into the general category of "how much have you shifted?"

First, if you have shifted completely and you can tell your SUDS for that issue is now a zero, you may want to consider that issue resolved. However, this is also an opportunity to explore it a little bit to really make sure it's resolved, and that there aren't any related issues waiting to be tapped on as well. For example, if I were working with someone on their fear of spiders, and they had gotten to a zero for seeing a spider, I would ask them to consider what it would be like to see a spider moving, or walking away from them, or walking toward them. Each of those could be a related aspects that should probably be addressed at the same time while the focus is on "fear of spiders." It is also an example of "taking a problem apart into its component pieces and then dealing with each one individually."

Second, if you have noticed a shift but your SUDS is not yet at a zero (or at least pretty darn close) then I would definitely recommend doing some more tapping on the issue. And I'd also include "...this remaining..." in the Setup and Reminder Phrases. Sometimes persistence is required in order to really "finish things off," but it is well worth it in my experience.

I noticed an initial shift, but now I'm stuck...

If you have noticed a shift initially, but are kind of stuck with the SUDS rating not changing much, there are several things to consider.

The initial thing to check in on, is have you shifted to another aspect of the issue, or even another issue altogether? Sometimes I've caught myself doing that without even noticing it to begin with. At times it appears that the issue that I'm tapping on is "so gone" that I don't even remember exactly what it was! Those are the times where it's a bit confusing and it points out even more clearly the value of writing the issue down, along with the SUDS rating, before starting to tap.

If that's not the case, then I'd do another round or two of tapping using the Setup Phrase and really saying it with emphasis while tapping on the KC. Sometimes we get stuck when there is some psychological reversal to getting over the issue and doing this, we can restart us down the path of progress.

The next thing I'd check in on is the definition of the issue. Sometimes we start to tackle a larger issue and make some progress, as indicated by a SUDS reduction, and then run into a brick wall. It may appear that EFT Tapping isn't working, but you may simply be trying to work on too many aspects at once. What I recommend is that you take a moment and see if you can break the issue down further into sub-components. For example, I would not try to address a "fear of flying" by tapping on "fear of flying" but rather I'd try to break it down into its components. In my experience, a "fear of flying" may have sub-components like, fear of heights, motion of the airplane, not knowing what's going to happen, not being in control (of the aircraft or situation) and possibly even the smells associated with jet engine exhaust that is sometimes around airports. There could even be sub-components that are associated with memories of movies, television shows, or news reports. These sub-components will vary from person to person, and what I would recommend is starting with whatever feeling is "most in your face" in terms of SUDS intensity. Once the SUDS intensity of that one reduces and falls away, I'd start tapping on the next most intense or "in your face" aspect that shows up. It's likely that something like this will have many aspects and each of them should be considered and tapped on individually as part of an overall set of tapping that is done in order to alleviate the overall issue or symptoms.

The other way I'd approach this is to check in and see if there is a reason why it is not "safe to get over the problem" that our subconscious could be using to hold onto the problem. A big part of the job of our subconscious is to "keep us safe" and it will sometimes object strongly to things that it perceives as a threat to our safety. And those "threats" may be something that a 4-year-old would think is a threat, but not an adult. So they may seem somewhat odd at times. For example, if you find yourself starting to get a Migraine Headache when the time to go visit your overbearing mother-in-law is drawing near, then your subconscious may be trying to "keep you safe" by preventing you from being subjected to that situation. Kind of a crude example, I know, but it illustrates the point. The issue (or at least the trigger) may not be where you expect it to be and it may not be obvious at all. Sometimes these things take a bit of detective work in order to find the "real issue" to tap on.

What should I do if I don't notice a shift?

The first thing that I would consider is the problem or issue definition to begin with. Is it too broad or general?

What I recommend is that you take a moment and see if you can break the issue down further into sub-components. For example, I would not try to address a "fear of flying" by tapping on "fear of flying" but rather I'd try to break it down into its components. I also probably wouldn't start out by tapping on "this Migraine" but rather take a moment to really home in on the SUDS, Character, and Location. In my experience a Migraine will likely have sub-components, just like a "fear of flying" may have many sub-components such as, fear of heights, motion of the airplane, the feeling of turbulence, claustrophobia, not knowing what's going to happen, not being in control (of the aircraft or situation) and possibly even the smells associated with jet engine exhaust that is sometimes around airports. There could even be sub-components that are associated with memories of movies, television shows, or news reports.

Tapping Frequently Asked Questions

For a Migraine, or any physical issue, I prefer to view these sub-components through the lens of Character and Location. For example in the description:

"A dull and throbbing pain slightly behind and above the inside edge of your left eye with a SUDS intensity rating of a 5. Tension in the muscles of your scalp, with a general SUDS intensity of a 3, but it is stronger on the left side above your ear with a SUDS of 4 in that area. Your vision is slightly "off" but full blown auras haven't started yet so it has a SUDS of 2."

The pain has a "dull and throbbing" Character, while the Character associated with the scalp is "muscle tension," and the Character associated with the vision symptom is, "slightly off." The Location of the pain is "slightly behind and above the inside edge of your left eye," while there are two Locations noted for the muscle tension - "the scalp" in general, and "on the scalp on the left side above your ear." The Location of the vision issue would obviously be the eyes. However if only one eye, or only one section of your vision was "slightly off," then that should be noted as the Location.

These sub-components will vary from person to person, and what I would recommend is starting with whatever feeling is "most in your face" in terms of SUDS intensity. Once the SUDS intensity of that one reduces and falls away, I'd start tapping on the next most intense, or "in your face," aspect that shows up. It's likely that something like this will have several aspects and each of them should be considered, and tapped on individually as part of an overall set of tapping`.

The second thing I'd consider is being persistent. I'd do another round or two of tapping using the Setup Phrase and really saying it with emphasis, while tapping on the KC. Sometimes we get stuck when there is some psychological reversal to getting over the issue and doing this can restart us down the path of progress.

A third approach would be to check in and see if there is a reason why it is "not safe to get over the problem," that our subconscious could be using to hold onto the issue. A big part of the job of our subconscious is to "keep us safe" and it will sometimes object strongly to things that it perceives as threats to our safety. And those "threats" may be something that a 4-year-old would think is a threat, but not an adult. So they may seem somewhat odd sometimes.

For example if you find yourself starting to get a Migraine Headache when the time to go visit your overbearing mother-in-law is drawing near, then your subconscious may be trying to "keep you safe" by preventing you from being subjected to that situation. Kind of a crude example, I know, but it illustrates the point. The issue (or at least the trigger) may not be where you expect it to be and it may not be obvious at all. Sometimes these things take a bit of detective work in order to find the "real issue" to tap on.

And finally, if none of the other suggestions have created a result, I'd do a at least three rounds of full EFT Tapping on "Even though I'm not making progress tapping on this issue, I deeply and completely love and accept myself, and I'm open to the possibility that whatever is blocking my progress will become obvious to me, so I can address it." I would go through the Setup three times making sure to tap on the KC while saying this with emphasis. Then I would go through at least three rounds of tapping being sure to tap on all of the regular EFT Tapping points while using a Reminder Phrase like, "This Hidden Block." Then I would pause, get quiet for a moment, and see if an answer pops into my head. More often than not, this procedure will lead to some kind of insight that starts you moving forward again. And the insight may come later in the day, or even in the next few days. By telling your subconscious that you are open to the possibility of the answer showing up, you are asking it to deliver the answer to you. Sometimes it takes a while because we are so busy, and our heads are so full all the time, that the subconscious has trouble finding an "open slot" to put the information into so it can get your attention! Give it time and space and you'll likely be surprised at what shows up!

How do I know when I'm "done" tapping?

On the surface, the most obvious answer is that you have "shifted completely" and you can tell that your SUDS, for that issue, is now a zero. You may be tempted to consider that issue resolved. However, this is also an opportunity to explore it a little bit to really make sure it's resolved and that there aren't any related issues waiting to be tapped on as well.

For example, if I were working with someone on their fear of spiders, and they had gotten to a zero for seeing a spider, I would ask them to consider what it would be like to see a spider moving, or walking away from them, or walking toward them. Each of those could be related aspects that should probably be addressed at the same time while the focus is on "fear of mice." It is also an example of "taking a problem apart into its component pieces and then dealing with each one individually."

The other thing that I'd suggest is to see if you can "test it" to check if the issue is really gone. Start by VIVIDLY imagining the situation. Exaggerate sounds, sights, and feelings as you imagine it. If that does not create a response then I'd suggest trying to SAFELY test it in the real world if you can.

For example, it is one thing to sit in your living room and "tap away" your fear of heights and assume that the issue is resolved because you have no negative response when you imagine a situation that would have previously triggered the fear. It is an entirely different thing to actually be standing on the observation deck of the Empire State Building looking over the edge of the railing, and enjoying the view! Putting yourself SAFELY in the situation is a good test of whether or not the issue is resolved. You need to take responsibility for yourself and your safety, so "sneak up on" the things you are testing. And if you do start to get a response as you're testing, in the real world, stop and do some more tapping on what comes up for you before you do any further testing or approach the situation closer. There is no need to "grit your teeth and push through it," because with EFT Tapping you can release the issue much more gently. Sure, it may take a few more rounds of tapping, but in the end it is well worth it to have emotional freedom from that issue!

How can I be even more effective with EFT Tapping?

My first suggestion is to use EFT Tapping more often. There are often little annoyances or upsets that show up during the day. While we can often let them go over the next few hours or days, by applying EFT Tapping to the upset, we can release it much more quickly, as well as benefit from the generalization effect that often goes along with tapping.

What Gary Craig noticed over his many years of working with tapping and teaching it to people, is that there is a generalization effect. For example, if there were 100 trees in "the emotional upset forest of your past" you probably won't have to address all 100 with EFT

Tapping. You may find that after dealing with 10, or 20, or 30 that the whole forest starts to collapse. That's definitely one of the "side benefits" of investing your time in tapping. And tapping on the little things certainly helps to dig away at the roots of some of those trees so they collapse that much faster.

Another suggestion is to ask the question "Is there an earlier similar situation to this one? Often times that question will lead to the memory of an earlier time when something similar happened that laid the foundation on which the current issue sits. Just like with a real building, if you knock out the foundation, the rest of the building will collapse. I always try to discover, and go after, the "earlier similar" incidents whenever I can find them. Tapping on those issues will also help to bring down even more "trees in the forest" that much faster.

In a similar vein, stepping back and looking at the tapping issue from an entirely different viewpoint, will often provide insights and additional tapping fodder, or paths to success, in eliminating the issues. Checking in on questions like, "What would I lose, or gain?" or even, "Who would be upset if I did or didn't achieve my goal?" can often lead to surprising insights and tappable issues.

21-Ways To Get Even Better Results...

As I have been finishing up the last steps to complete the publication of this book, I have also been creating some great new content that is focused on 21 ways to get even better results with EFT Tapping. This information will help show you some of my personal favorite tips, tricks, and secrets for being even more effective when you use EFT Tapping. I am also including some specific ways that you can apply EFT Tapping in order to create an even better life for yourself.

Be sure to check it out at:

http://tapping4.us/21ways

Frequently Asked Questions For Migraine Headaches

In anticipation that people will skip around within this section, I have included the "check with a qualified medical practitioner" comment in several of the answers. There is some additional repetition of comments within this section so that each of the answers can stand by itself and be complete.

It hurts so bad that I don't want to physically tap, is there another way?

Yes, there are several suggestions I can share in this situation.

First, you can "touch and breathe" instead of tapping. Simply touch the tapping location and breathe in and out one time before moving on to the next point and doing the same thing. What this does is place your attention on the spot while you go through a breathing cycle and saying the Reminder Phrase out loud (or even mentally saying it if that's all you can do.)

You can take this to the next level by imagining tapping on the spots while imagining saying the Reminder Phrase out loud. It may not be as effective as physically tapping or touching the spots, but again if that's the best you can do, it's the best you can do. And you may find that after you've taken the edge off it, that you are able to move to physically touching or tapping on the locations as the next step on your road to relief.

Another thing that you can try is to watch a video of someone tapping and substitute the words for "your issue" for the ones used in the video. Again it would be beneficial to vividly imagine that you are doing the tapping on your body in order get the best result. If that takes the edge off for you then perhaps you can start physically tapping along while focusing on your issue with your words.

My child's pain is so intense that they won't let me help by tapping on them. Is there another way to help them with EFT?

(Please note that while I focused the explanation on a working with a child, this may work equally as well with an adult.)

Yes, there are several suggestions I can share in this situation.

First, you can help them by using the "touch and breathe" technique instead of tapping. Simply touch the tapping location and have them breathe in and out one time before moving on to the next tapping point and doing the same thing. This will place their attention on the spot while they go through a breathing cycle. You can say the Reminder Phrase out loud for them so they stay focused on the issue. And you can tell them that they can mentally substitute their description of the issue (or Location, and Character of the pain) while you are doing this. Eventually, once it takes the edge off, they may start volunteering the words, and descriptions, out-loud for you.

If they won't let you even touch them, you can try taking this to the next level by having them imagining tapping on the spots while you are naming the tapping location and saying the Reminder Phrase out loud. It may not be as effective as physically tapping or touching the spots, but again if that's the best you can do in the moment, it's the best you can do. And you may find that after this has taken the edge off it, that you are able to move to physically touching or tapping on them as the next step on their road to relief.

Another thing that you can try is to have them watch you as you are tapping on yourself for their issue. As strange as this sounds, it can be the start of the road to relief. This is especially true if you tap into your intuition and go with the flow of what you feel, or at least imagine it would be like in their situation, and tap using the words that come to mind to describe their situation. And when it comes to kids and pain, remember that it might be really scary to them to be in that much pain too, so address that fear if you think it would apply.

Other Headache Tips And Tricks...

I wanted to share a couple other tricks that I've run across. Try these out sometime and see how they work for you.

Base of the skull tapping

A few years ago, a friend of a friend watched an early Migraine tapping video that I put together. She reported back that the technique didn't help her as much as expected until she added in another tapping point. She added tapping around the bony ridge area at the back of the base of her skull, and once she included that, she noticed increased symptom relief.

In the message she sent me, she also mentioned that when she was a little girl, and had a headache, her mother would rub and tap that area at the base of her skull. It's unclear to me if that's a "real tapping point," which is quite possible since there are acupuncture energy meridians that run through that area, or if that was simply "her spot" as a result of her childhood experience.

My point in including this here, is that not only do I want to share all of my "secrets" with you, but to also point out that each of may have some personal resources that we've forgotten about. Think back through your personal history and you may find a gold nugget like that waiting for you too.

"Headache Point" on the hand

Several times I've heard about "the headache point" on the hand. It is in the middle of the fleshy web between you thumb and the side of your hand. (In the vicinity of the white triangle in the photo below.) This is the muscle that moves the thumb closer to the side of your hand. While it is often very uncomfortable to do, some people have reported getting substantial relief from headaches by pinching and rubbing the muscle in that web.

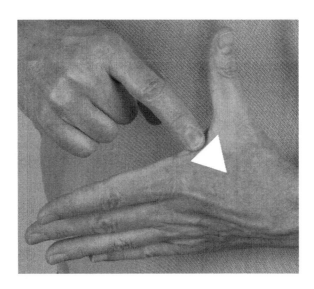

Other Headache Tips And Tricks

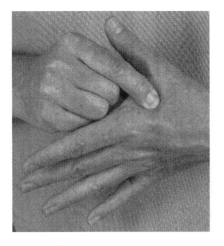 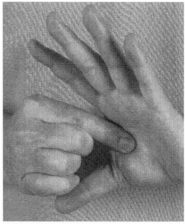

I've heard that it may be more effective on one hand or the other, so you may want to try rubbing and massaging that muscle on both hands. If one is more tender and painful than the other, it is said that's the one to work on the most.

This is sometimes referred to as "Trigger Point Therapy" in the massage world. As strange as it sounds, it is thought that there is a "headache Trigger Point" in that area, and by applying pressure to the trigger point (by squeezing it) the trigger point may eventually release, and along with it, release at least some of the headache pain.

The idea here is to work the muscle and relax it by pinching it between your thumb and index finger of the other hand. You may want to try massaging that whole (white triangle) area and the muscles underneath.

Section 3:
Tips, Tricks, And Secrets For Using EFT Tapping

In this section I want to share with you a number of tips, tricks, and secrets that I use with EFT Tapping. These are simple little things that once you know about them you can often get better and faster results with your EFT Tapping.

Floor-To-Ceiling Eye Roll Shortcut

In Gary Craig's original training DVD's he shows a shortcut technique that often times can be very effective in releasing the last little bit of an issue in less time than it takes to do a full round of tapping. He would typically apply it when the SUDS level had dropped to a one or a two.

The "floor-to-ceiling eye roll" is done by holding your head still, and starting with your eyes looking hard down toward the floor, and then slowly, over about 6 seconds or so, rolling them up to looking at the ceiling

Fast Migraine Headache Relief With EFT Tapping

(all while holding your head still) while tapping continuously on "the 9-gamut spot."

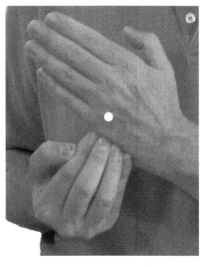

"The 9-gamut spot" is on the back of your hand just behind the knuckles where your "ring finger" and "baby finger" meet your hand. There is kind of a groove there that you tap on continuously while doing the floor-to-ceiling-eye-roll.

Next time you find your SUDS intensity down at a 1 or a 2, give it a try and see what you think. Sometimes it works well with just one round; other times it takes a couple of tries. If the floor-to-ceiling-eye-roll is not resolving the issue and bringing the SUDS to a zero, then go ahead and do a regular round of EFT Tapping instead.

As an enhancement to this book, I created two video showing the Floor-To-Ceiling Eye Roll more clearly than can be done with words photos alone. You can see the first Floor-To-Ceiling Eye Roll video here:

http://tapping4.us/eyeroll.

The second Floor-To-Ceiling Eye Roll video is a more close-up shot where you can see my eye position more clearly, and it can be found here:

http://tapping4.us/eyeroll2.

You can find a complete list of videos and other internet content in the Resources section.

Finger Tapping Points

When Gary originally created EFT he included five additional tapping points on the hand they are less commonly used today. However, they are good ones to know about, especially as alternative tapping points. In addition to the 9-Gamut point described above, there are tapping point on the thumb, index finger, middle finger, and little finger. (The meridian on the ring finger is picked up at another location on the body.)

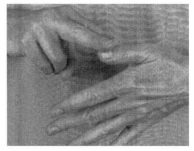

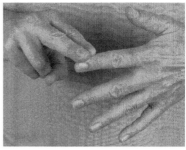

You might try tapping on these points in addition to, or as a replacement for, other tapping points. This could be particularly useful when you have Migraine Headache symptoms and do not want to tap on your face or head. Instead, try using the finger points. The procedure is the same – tapping while

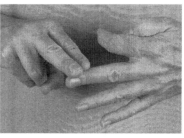

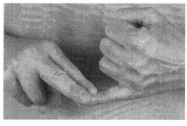

focusing on the issue and saying the Reminder Phrase – as with the regular EFT Tapping shown throughout this book.

Finger tapping, or even rubbing or massaging the finger points, could also be used in public when you want to be more discrete, or otherwise hide the tapping you are doing. Simply focus on the issue, or the Character, and Location in the case of physical pain, and "think out loud" the Reminder Phrase while rubbing or tapping on your fingers.

As an enhancement to this book, I created a video showing the tapping locations on the fingers of the hand more clearly than can be done with words photos alone. You can see the finger tapping locations video here:

`http://tapping4.us/hand.`

You can find a complete list of videos and other internet content in the Resources section.

Mental Tapping

You can do it anywhere, anytime, without anyone knowing what you're doing. When physical tapping is "not possible" or would be disruptive, you can try vividly imagining doing the tapping instead. When you're doing this for Migraine symptoms, be sure to focus on the Character, and Location while mentally tapping. The key is to imagine tapping on each point as vividly as possible. Closing your eyes may enhance your focus and reduce distractions while you mentally tap on each point. You can often get results in minutes with mental tapping. It may be a bit slower than physical tapping, but it is often still very effective.

Mental tapping can also provide a way around the embarrassment of tapping in public. If you find that mental tapping isn't working as well as you'd like, an alternative would be to excuse yourself from the situation and go tap somewhere by yourself. The bathroom is always a great "hiding place" for tapping.

Public tapping without embarrassment

Another few words about: How can I tap "in public" without feeling embarrassed? Whenever that question comes up, my first response is always: Tap on "feeling embarrassed about tapping in public!" Then, after everyone gets over the "Yeah, DUH!" moment, I also go on to say that instead of physically tapping, you can vividly imagine tapping on the points like we just discussed.

As a side note: in the book Entangled Minds by Dean Radin, PhD., he includes information on studies that show the brain cannot tell the difference between REAL or vividly imagined events. Entangled Minds is available through Amazon.com:

http://tapping4.us/eminds

You CAN tap with your mind by vividly imagining your fingers tapping on each point in succession, and be able to get the issue to greatly lessen, if not be completely resolved! Be persistent and keep at it.

Free Online Resources

There are lots of tapping resources that can be found online. There are even many tapping videos on YouTube. Because EFT is so easy to learn, many people like to share it with others. Unfortunately, sometimes this "second-hand EFT" is incorrect or can be misleading. As a result, you will want to be cautious in selecting what to pay attention to.

My recommendation is that you start with EmoFree.com – which was Gary Craig's "official" EFT site. Gary has retired the original EmoFree.com site along with all of its user-supplied mini-case-studies. He has restructured EmoFree.com to feature the Official EFT Tutorials that he created. I know that he is interested in "keeping the technology pure," so to speak, and has some differences of opinion about the way some people have modified EFT Tapping. I trust Gary, especially since he created EFT and has obviously been using it and testing it longer than anyone else on the planet!

It is unclear if Gary has an "official" repository for the content that was on EmoFree.com but when I did a search for "Brad Reed helps with the fear of flying" I did find a site (www.danachivers-eft.com) that appears to have cloned much of Gary's original EmoFree.com content. That could be a great resource because the original site had hundreds of topics catalogued there and it could give you ideas for what's possible with EFT Tapping.

I did a Google search for:
```
migraine site:www.danachivers-eft.com
```
and Google found 194 results! (That is a Google search in the form <search_term> site:<website_to_search>)

There are lots of tapping script ideas and Setup Phrase examples in the articles.

The bottom line is that this is an Extensive archive that includes thousands of pages of great content gathered by Gary as case studies and examples of applying EFT in everyday real life situations. You can use the case studies to find additional phrases for tapping, as well as seeing how other people have addressed their individual issues with EFT Tapping.

Tapping Journal

Use a simple $0.99 notebook to keep track of your Migraine symptom's Character, Location, and SUDS. Not only will this help you in the beginning when you are new to EFT Tapping for Migraine symptoms, but by taking some extra notes about your day (what you ate, stress level, weather changes, etc.) you may find some common themes that you can address, either with EFT Tapping or through other means (like removing it from your diet.)

And once you start using EFT Tapping to address issues beyond Migraine symptoms, not only can you use your tapping journal to capture topics for future tapping sessions, but tracking your progress will encourage you to tap more, as well as reminding you of how much progress you've made. When you run across topics to tap on, write them down. Not only can you use it when you are actively tapping, but you can also note things to address later if you don't have time to tap on them in the moment. Use it to record "areas for exploration" when you're not quite ready to "dig in" to them, but you don't want to forget them later.

Saying it like it is: Be politically INcorrect with your phrasing

Be "Politically Incorrect" with your phrasing so you can get deeper results faster! This is especially true when you're focused on reducing your stress level with an eye toward Migraine symptom prevention. There are many times in our lives where we censor ourselves, and what we really want to say, in order to be politically correct, or socially acceptable in the situation. However, when you're tapping, especially by yourself, say what you really feel while you're tapping! Express yourself!! Reconnect with your Inner Sailor - go ahead, and swear up a storm! It may not have ever been safe for you to fully express yourself and how you were really feeling. Now is the time to really get in touch with that so that you can finally let it go! There is no need to be "Politically Correct" when tapping, especially if you're by yourself.

For example, if you're working on trying to get into better shape, don't waste your time tapping on "I don't like to exercise" when the truth is that you feel "Exercise is a pain in the ass!" Tap on that instead! It's YOUR TRUTH after all!

You are likely to get even better results if you really get into the emotion of how you feel! You can't help but tune into the issue when you are "venting about it." You are likely to start out "heated" and end up feeling a bit silly! – especially when you are venting in what I call a "tap-and-bitch session." This shift from heated to silly is a good thing because it indicates that things really ARE shifting!

A quick story here. Not long ago I was REALLY, REALLY, (did I mention REALLY!!) mad and frustrated with myself for an ongoing situation. The frustration had been smoldering the entire morning, and when I finally climbed into the shower, I couldn't stand it anymore and really unleashed venomously on myself, WHILE I WAS TAPPING. It was a "tap-and-bitch session" in the shower. I was actually shocked at how quickly the SUDS intensity and my viewpoint shifted. I don't think I had ever admitted to myself how much anger and frustration I had toward myself about this issue. But I certainly did that day. Because I was totally in the feeling there was no question that I was "tuned into the issue" and in a matter of moments there was a huge drop in the anger and frustration level. I don't think I even got past the 3rd or 4th point, after doing a bunch of tapping on the KC and venting about the frustration, before it shifted from "about a 15" down to about a 7, and then it continued to drop rapidly from there. In the end, I had to admit to myself, that even though I didn't like the way things were going, I really was doing the best that I could ... in the moment.

That's something that we lose sight of sometimes – we really are doing the best we can in the moment, even if it may not look like it. As proof of that, when was the last time that you chose to do a mediocre job of something that you care about or wanted results from? I'm betting that you really do the "best" that you can <u>in the moment</u> pretty much all the time (even if it may not look like it to an outsider.)

When it comes to shifting your response to external (and internal) stressors, consider adding a final round of EFT Tapping, starting with tapping on the KC while saying "Even though I may not like what's going on, I deeply and completely love and accept myself, and I acknowledge that we really are doing the best we can, even though it may not look like it!" Then tap through a couple of rounds alternating between the Reminder Phrases, "doing the best we can" and "even though it may not look like it" as you tap. What I've found for myself, it that this puts a very nice finishing touch on this kind of tapping round, and generally reduces my stress level another notch.

Tap-And-Bitch

It's the FAST way to release upset, anger, and frustration when it happens. This is a great way to reduce your stress level and maybe prevent Migraine symptoms from showing up. When "life gets crappy" and you have something to "bitch about," simply "<u>tell the story</u>" of what you're upset about, WHILE TAPPING THE WHOLE TIME! Keep tapping through all the points, over and over again, until you "take the emotional charge off it" and it is not so upsetting. Even better, keep tapping until you're truly neutral about it. Being "neutral" may show up as being bored with the story or the topic.

Parents – This works great with kids, and their little "boo-boo" injuries! Have them tell the story of what happened while tapping on them. "Tap-and-tell" is the kid appropriate version of "Tap-and-bitch."

I want to share with you something I witnessed myself that made me a believer in this approach. Jennifer's son was about 5-years-old when he fell out of a tree he was climbing. After we had checked him out to be sure that the only damage was to his pride, we asked him what had happened. Through his tears, and of course using his wonderful 5-year-old logic, he explained how he blamed falling out of the tree on his brother, who was inside watching him out the window at the time. During this explanation, Jen started tapping on his EFT points while he told the story. She asked him to go over it several times as she continued tapping on him. Pretty soon, after maybe the third retelling, he said he was completely bored with it and asked if could he go back and climb the tree again! The really cool part about this was there was no hesitation to "get back on the horse that threw him" so to speak, like so many kids exhibit after a traumatic fall like that. To this day, he still has no fear when it comes to climbing in trees! For me, this is further proof of the power of tapping in the moment to help eliminate any stuck trauma that could "leave a mark" for the rest of your life.

Because I know this is such a powerful strategy that can be used to release your emotional upset fast, I even created a website that focuses on this method. You can find it at:

http://www.TapAndBitch.com

When you enter your name and email address in the box in the upper right-hand corner of the site, you will be sent access to a free, 23-minute video that I created called The EFT Quick Start Video Learning System. I would strongly recommend that you check it out. (Not to be crude or offense, but "TapAndComplain.com" simply doesn't have the same impact and isn't nearly as memorable either.)

Borrowing Benefits

You can "get your tapping work done" while focused on someone else tapping on their issue. "Borrowing the Benefits" is done by tapping along with someone else addressing their issue. It sounds somewhat strange, but Gary Craig has witnessed how effective it is many times, and even demonstrates it in one of his training videos.

First, find a recording of someone tapping on their issue. You could use the Migraine tapping example videos or other tapping videos that I reference in this book. You could even search YouTube for an EFT Tapping video that is similar to whatever you're addressing.

Then choose a symptom, or an issue that's bugging you, and give it a SUDS rating – or note the SUDS, Character, and Location if it is a physical issue. It can be completely unrelated to the issue being addressed in the recording. Then tap along with the recording while focusing ON THEIR ISSUE AND USING THEIR PHRASING. When you are finished with the tap along, re-rate your issue and it is highly likely that it will have shifted a bit and may have dropped at least a few SUDS points too.

Yes, with this method you really can tap on something completely different and unrelated to your issue, and likely still get fabulous results! By bringing your issue to mind before tapping along with someone else, your subconscious will "apply" the tapping to the item you've chosen to address before you started tapping along. The subconscious mind is an amazing thing!

You can also use this to help someone else, like a child, by walking them through the process along with you. You could even be the one doing the tapping and they can follow along. Before you start, you could ask something like "If you had a magic wand that could make this tapping apply to anything, what would it be?" That would get the child focused on the issue – even if they don't want to tell you what it is! Next, simply ask them if it would be OK if that happened while they tapped along with you, and then start tapping on "your issue" even if you have to make it up!

You may not get results as fast as if you addressed the issue head-on, but hey, if you can drop a few SUDS points while tapping along with someone else, and you don't have to "confront your issues," take it!

Conclusion

We have covered a lot of ground in this book. Not only have you had an opportunity to learn the basics of EFT Tapping and experience a couple of tapping script demonstrations, but the material and approaches presented here for addressing Migraine symptoms are probably unlike anything you've seen before.

In addition to learning the basic EFT Tapping mechanics (SUDS, Setup, Tapping – EB, SE, UE, UN, CH, CB, UA, Top) you have seen how you can apply EFT Tapping to Migraine Headache symptoms as well as other more general topics. I'm confident that by participating in the EFT Tapping demonstrations presented in this book, that you have had an opportunity to experience a shift for yourself. Hopefully, you will never need them, but information on common difficulties in applying EFT Tapping provides quite a few nuggets of wisdom that may help you move forward again rapidly once applied.

The material covered in the second section on applying EFT Tapping for fast Migraine Headache relief should have provided you with more than adequate information to tackle your next set of Migraine Headache symptoms. The Example Tapping Script Walk-Through is a reference that I suggest you revisit whenever you need a refresher, or you can even use it verbatim as a starting point for dealing with your next Migraine Headache symptoms.

The section on Using EFT Tapping to address Migraine Headache Triggers provides unique content found nowhere else, and can provide a solid foundation from which to explore addressing Migraine symptom triggers with an eye toward their reduction or even elimination.

The Tapping FAQ has lots of valuable information that includes guidance about what to do when you do, or do not, notice a shift from tapping. This information in particular should become second nature to you as you gain more experience with EFT Tapping – both for Migraine symptoms and when applying it to other topics.

The final major section on Tips, Tricks, and Secrets for using EFT Tapping includes some of my favorites, along with links to some specific resources that I use and recommend personally.

I trust that you found your investment in reading this book to pay very high dividends, and it will be a resource that you can "tap" into for the rest of your life. I know that once I found EFT Tapping and started applying it to various aspects of my life, I have never looked back when it comes to the continuous progress that I've made in creating a better life for myself. I wish you the same success!

I'd like to make request of you now that you've read this book, please leave a review on Amazon:

http://tapping4.us/review-migraine.

Resources

Videos

- **EFT Tapping Locations video:** http://tapping4.us/tappingspots
- **Chocolate Craving Demo video:** http://tapping4.us/chocolatedemo
- **Gary Craig's Constricted Breathing demonstration:** http://tapping4.us/breathing
- **Migraine EFT Tapping Script Walk Through video:** http://tapping4.us/migrainewalkthru
- **Migraine Tapping Fast Start video:** http://tapping4.us/migrainefaststart
- **Floor-To-Ceiling Eye Roll video:** http://tapping4.us/eyeroll
- **Close-up Floor-To-Ceiling Eye Roll video:** http://tapping4.us/eyeroll2
- **Finger tapping locations video:** http://tapping4.us/hand

Downloadable EFT Tapping Cheat Sheets

- **EFT Tapping on a Page:**
  http://tapping4.us/cheat-sheet

- **EFT Tapping on a Page – Migraine Edition:**
  http://tapping4.us/migraine-book-cheat-sheet

Scholarly Research

- **Dr. David Feinstein:**
  http://tapping4.us/research-feinstein

- **EFT Universe - Research Links:**
  http://tapping4.us/research-universe

From the Author, Brad Reed

- **21-Ways To Get Even Better Results With EFT Tapping!**
  http://tapping4.us/21ways

- **Amazon Author Central page**
  http://tapping4.us/authorcentral

- **The Secret For Law Of Attraction – What the gurus aren't telling you:**
  http://tapping4.us/tsfloa-dvd

- **Release Your Emotional Upset Fast:**
  http://TapAndBitch.com

- **The Author's Blog:**
  http://tapping4.us/bradsblog

- **Connect with the author on social media**
  http://tapping4.us/social

A limited number of private tapping sessions are available. For pricing and to request a session, please email:

> WithEFTtapping@gmail.com

Other Resources

- **Entangled Minds by Dean Radin, PhD.**
  http://tapping4.us/eminds

Please leave a review of this book on Amazon.com

http://tapping4.us/review-migraine

About the Author

Brad Reed was trained as an Electrical Engineer back in the 1980's. While he loved the logic and fun that came from designing electronic circuits for a test equipment manufacturer, he also found that what he really enjoyed was working with people to solve their problems. Once he left the design bench, he never looked back, and was always helping people in one way or another. At work he helped people with the technology that was part of his job. Outside of work he was fascinated by people and what influences their behavior. This curiosity led to the pursuit of a variety of "self-help and healing modalities" on the road to improving not only his life, but also the lives of others.

It was when he found EFT Tapping that the real excitement began. Not only was EFT created by Gary Craig, a Stanford University trained engineer, but it was the first modality he found that could regularly and predictably produce consistent results for a wide variety of people and issues. And on top of that, it was easy to use and easy to teach to other people.

Brad jumped at the chance when the opportunity to study with Gary Craig presented itself, and he spent multiple weekends under Gary's tutelage in various live classes. He also invested in Gary's video training and studied it extensively. Not only did this study improve his tapping skills, but it also led to earning his EFT Cert-1 through the only program recommended by Gary shortly before his retirement.

In addition to the "EFT book learning" that has honed his skills, the exposure to a wide variety of "self-help and healing modalities" has given him a greater depth of understanding and perspective than is present in many tapping practitioners. In addition because of his engineering background and being steeped in observation and problem solving, his clients have told him repeatedly that he brings unique insights to addressing and resolving their issues. This comment is particularly common among the tapping practitioners he works with occasionally.

While this may be his first published written work (outside of the Electrical Engineering realm) it most certainly won't be his last. There are plans for a long list of ...With EFT Tapping books that address a variety of topics. Be sure to look up his latest Kindle publications on Amazon.com through his Amazon Author Central page:

http://tapping4.us/authorcentral

And don't miss his DVD, *The Secret For Law Of Attraction – What the gurus aren't telling you*, available through Amazon.com:

http://tapping4.us/tsfloa-dvd

This DVD shows how to apply EFT Tapping to release the self-sabotage that limits our success in applying the Law Of Attraction. It was created in

About The Author

response to the hype around "The Secret" which resulted in many people being disillusioned because of their lack of success with the Law Of Attraction. Little did they know what the real roadblock was to their success or how to change it. Watch the DVD to learn those insights and how to apply EFT Tapping in your life.

A limited number of private, one-on-one, sessions are available to work directly with individual clients. If you would like to schedule one, please contact Brad by Email at:

`WithEFTtapping@gmail.com.`

Manufactured by Amazon.ca
Bolton, ON